Cases in
Nephrology

Cases in
Nephrology

Editor

Muhammad Rafiqul Alam MBBS MD FCPS
Professor of Nephrology and Ex Pro vice Chancellor
Bangabandhu Sheikh Mujib Medical University
President, Bangladesh Renal Association
President, Association of Physicians of Bangladesh
Vice President, Society of Organ Transplantation, Bangladesh
Member, Editorial board of Bangladesh Renal Journal

Forewords
Harun-Ur-Rashid
Md Sharfuddin Ahmed

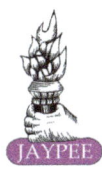

JAYPEE BROTHERS MEDICAL PUBLISHERS
The Health Sciences Publisher
New Delhi | London

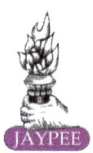

JAYPEE **Jaypee Brothers Medical Publishers (P) Ltd**

Headquarters
EMCA House
23/23-B, Ansari Road, Daryaganj
New Delhi 110 002, India
Landline: +91-11-23272143, +91-11-23272703
+91-11-23282021, +91-11-23245672
E-mail: jaypee@jaypeebrothers.com

Corporate Office
Jaypee Brothers Medical Publishers (P) Ltd.
4838/24, Ansari Road, Daryaganj
New Delhi 110 002, India
Phone: +91-11-43574357
Fax: +91-11-43574314
E-mail: jaypee@jaypeebrothers.com

Overseas Office
JP Medical Ltd.
83, Victoria Street, London
SW1H 0HW (UK)
Phone: +44-20 3170 8910
E-mail: info@jpmedpub.com

EU GPSR Authorised Representative
Logos Europe, 9 rue Nicolas Poussin
17000, La Rochelle, France
Phone: +33 (0) 6 67 93 73 78
E-mail: Contact@logoseurope.eu

Website: www.jaypeebrothers.com
Website: www.jaypeedigital.com

Inquiries for bulk sales may be solicited at: jaypee@jaypeebrothers.com

Cases in Nephrology / *Muhammad Rafiqul Alam*

First Edition: **2023**

ISBN: 978-93-5465-957-7

Dedicated to

My Students
They are Like my Children.

FOREWORD

Internal medicine has got many distinct subspecialties; Nephrology is one of them. Postgraduate courses in Nephrology is conducted by Bangabandhu Sheikh Mujib Medical University and also by Bangladesh College of Physicians and Surgeons for a long time. More recently, medical officers are getting interested to obtain training in Nephrology and also to do postgraduate degrees in this specialty. However, there are always scarcity of recent textbooks of Nephrology in our region. In these circumstances, necessity of a short comprehensive problem oriented book is felt by trainee to acquire knowledge about Nephrology.

In this regard, I congratulate Professor Dr Muhammad Rafiqul Alam for compiling a short problem-oriented book in the form of case reports in Nephrology—"Cases in Nephrology". The author has discussed different nephrological cases, some of which are common and some are rare.

The way the cases are presented and discussed, will be helpful for medical officers, fellows, and residents in Nephrology all together.

I wish the book will get popularity among the readers.

Harun-Ur-Rashid
Founder President, Kidney Foundation, Bangladesh
ISN Pioneer Nephrologist of South Asia Region

FOREWORD

I feel privileged to write the foreword of the book *"Cases in Nephrology"* by Professor Dr Muhammad Rafiqul Alam. I used to encourage our faculties to get more and more involved in research activities, publish papers in reputed journals, and write book or chapter in a book. This enriches our knowledge armamentarium and at the same time, elevate the position of the University in the QS World University ranking.

My colleague, Dr Muhammad Rafiqul Alam, is involved in teaching nephrology discipline for a long time. In this book, Dr Muhammad Rafiqul Alam discussed thirty cases in a manner which will be helpful for fellows in nephrology, MD residents in nephrology for their preparation for fellowship examination, and MD Phase B residency examination. Fellows and residents in internal medicine will also be benefitted by the book.

I wish the book all success.

Md Sharfuddin Ahmed
Vice Chancellor
Bangabandhu Sheikh Mujib Medical University
Dhaka, Bangladesh

PREFACE

"Cases in Nephrology" is the compilation of the real-life clinical cases presented in the nephrology seminar room of the Bangabandhu Sheikh Mujib Medical University by the residents of MD Nephrology. Residents and fellows in Nephrology have to undergo summative examinations for obtaining their degree/diploma. Long case presentation and discussion is a very important part of their examination. Keeping this in mind, this book has been compiled.

Thirty cases have been discussed which I believe will help postgraduate trainees, residents, and fellows in Nephrology during their preparation for final examination.

Hopefully, deficits and mistakes will be corrected in future editions.

Finally, all praises go to Almighty!

Muhammad Rafiqul Alam

ACKNOWLEDGMENTS

Many people are involved in production of this book. It is difficult to mention all names. I would however like to thank Professor Dr Asia Khanam, Professor Dr Ferdousy Begum, Professor Sultana Gulshana Banu, Dr Shahjada Selim, Dr Mahbuba Shirin, and Dr Amit Bari and all the teachers, medical officers, residents of the department of Nephrology, Bangabandhu Sheikh Mujib Medical University, for their valuable contribution.

I owe particular thanks to my wife, my daughters, and my son-in-laws, granddaughters, and grandson who have provided emotional support and encouragement and patience during the writing process.

Finally, I must thank KM Haque, Md Towhidul Islam, and HM Arif Ur Rahman for the wonderful service in preparing the manuscript.

Finally, all praises go to Almighty!

Muhammad Rafiqul Alam

CONTENTS

Chapter 1:   Diabetic Nephropathy with Chronic Kidney Disease   1

Chapter 2:   Lupus Nephritis   6

Chapter 3:   Antineutrophil Cytoplasmic Antibody-positive
Glomerulonephritis   13

Chapter 4:   Post-transplant Thrombotic Microangiopathy   18

Chapter 5:   Transplantation in a Patient with Lower Urinary
Tract Abnormality   21

Chapter 6:   Preemptive Renal Transplantation   26

Chapter 7:   Acute Kidney Injury   31

Chapter 8:   Gitelman Syndrome   35

Chapter 9:   Renal Amyloidosis   38

Chapter 10: Down's Syndrome with Chronic Kidney Disease   43

Chapter 11: Continuous Ambulatory Peritoneal Dialysis
Peritonitis   46

Chapter 12: Wilson's Disease with Focal Segmental
Glomerulosclerosis   49

Chapter 13: Immunoglobulin M Nephropathy   53

Chapter 14: Membranoproliferative Glomerulonephritis   56

Chapter 15: Membranous Nephropathy   61

Chapter 16: Henoch–Schönlein Purpura Nephritis   66

Chapter 17: Alport Syndrome   72

Chapter 18: Lipomyelomeningocele with Tethered Cord
Syndrome, Neurogenic Bladder, CKD, and
Disseminated Tuberculosis   75

Chapter 19: Systemic Lupus Erythematous, Lupus Nephritis,
and Avascular Necrosis of Femoral Head   81

Chapter 20: **Membranous Nephropathy: Remission with Supportive Treatment**   85

Chapter 21: **Collagenofibrotic Glomerulopathy**   88

Chapter 22: **Cytomegalovirus Pneumonia in Kidney Transplant Patient**   93

Chapter 23: **Cellular Rejection in Renal Allograft Recipient**   97

Chapter 24: **Vascular Complication after Renal Transplantation**   105

Chapter 25: **Sepsis in a Renal Allograft Recipient**   112

Chapter 26: **Chronic Pyelonephritis due to Vesicoureteric Reflux, Secondary FSGS, Renal Abscess, and CKD**   115

Chapter 27: **Refractory Lupus Nephritis**   120

Chapter 28: **Systemic Amyloidosis Involving Kidney and Heart**   124

Chapter 29: **Myelodysplastic Syndrome and Nephrotic Syndrome**   127

Chapter 30: **Minimal Change Disease or Focal Segmental Glomerulosclerosis**   131

Index   135

Diabetic Nephropathy with Chronic Kidney Disease

INTRODUCTION

A 65-year-old female, known case of diabetes mellitus for 25 years, hypertension for 15 years, and ischemic heart disease for 3 years attended the outpatient department with the complaints of:
- Swelling of the body for 2 months
- Anorexia, nausea, and generalized weakness for 4 months
- Nonhealing ulcer on right foot with swelling and redness of left leg for 4 weeks
- Low-grade fever for 2 weeks

Initially, she was on diet and oral hypoglycemic drugs with poor diabetic control; for last 5 years, she is on insulin with history of three hypoglycemic episodes in last 6 months which has been managed at home. She is taking bisoprolol 5 mg OD and losartan 50 mg OD.

She gives history of laparoscopic cholecystectomy 10 years ago.

On physical examination, the patient was conscious and oriented. Face was puffy; pitting leg edema up to knee, there was redness and local rise of temperature in the left leg. There was an ulcer on the left great toe, which was small in size **(Fig. 1)**. Her blood pressure (BP) was 160/100 mm Hg (supine) and 130/80 mm Hg (standing), heart rate 84 bpm, peripheral pulses were palpable, features of peripheral neuropathy were present. All modalities of sensation decreased in gloves and stocking pattern and ankle jerk diminished. On fundoscopic examination, there was dot and blot hemorrhage and hard exudate in both eyes and also there is formation of neovessels, i.e., proliferative diabetic retinopathy (PDR) **(Figs. 2A and B)**. Cardiac and pulmonary auscultations were normal.

The urinalysis showed protein 3+, sugar +, white blood cell (WBC) 10–15/ high power field (HPF), and red blood cell (RBC) 1–2/HPF.

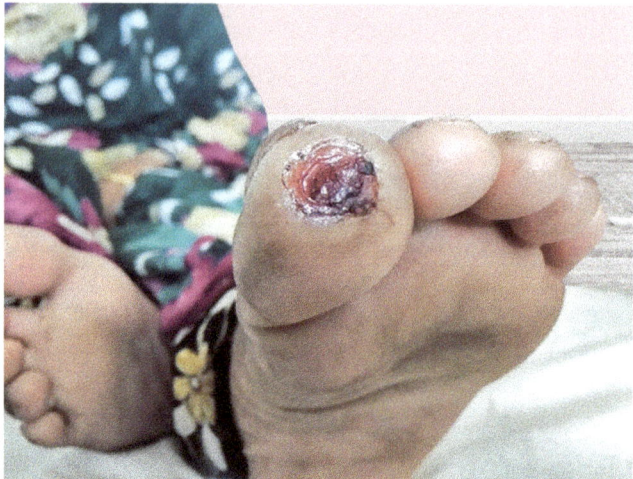

FIG. 1: Diabetic foot ulcer.

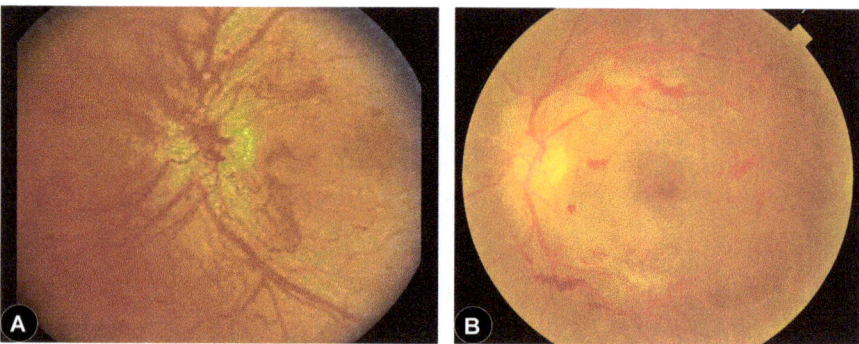

FIGS. 2A AND B: Diabetic proliferative retinopathy.

Complete blood count revealed hemoglobin (Hb) 10.2 g/dL erythrocyte sedimentation rate (ESR) 90 mm in 1st hour, WBC 16×10^9/L with neutrophil 87%, RBC 3.82×10^9/L, platelet count 340×10^9/L, serum creatinine 8.4 mg% (baseline was 5.4 mg%), serum sodium was 126 mmol/L, serum potassium was 4.8 mmol/L, serum calcium 1.6 mmol/L, serum inorganic phosphate 1.3 mmol/L, serum albumin 23 g/L, HbA1c 6%, spot urine albumin to creatinine ratio (UACR) was 5,212 mg/g. Ultrasonography of kidneys revealed diameter of right kidney 9.5 cm, left kidney 10.2 cm; increased cortical echogenicity with poor corticomedullary differentiation, fasting serum lipid profile showed total cholesterol 207 mg/dL, high-density lipoprotein (HDL) 34 mg/dL, low-density lipoprotein (LDL) 130 mg/dL, triglyceride 217 mg/dL, iron profile showed serum iron 29 µg/dL, total iron binding capacity (TIBC) 150 µg/dL, ferritin 466 ng/mL, transferrin saturation 19.3%, liver function and thyroid function was normal. Electrocardiography showed old anterior myocardial infarction.

Echocardiography showed hypokinesia of anterior wall and left ventricular ejection fraction 55%, culture of pus from foot ulcer showed growth of *Staphylococcus*. Urine culture showed no growth. After consultation with surgeon, cardiologist, diabetologist, and neurologist, treatment was initiated with antibiotics, debridement, and regular dressing of foot ulcer, statin, antiplatelet drugs along with insulin, losartan potassium, and bisoprolol. Hemodialysis was started through left femoral venous catheter. She was advised for arteriovenous fistula construction and maintenance hemodialysis twice in a week.

DISCUSSION

Diabetic nephropathy (DN) is the leading cause of chronic kidney disease worldwide.

Genetic, metabolic, immunologic, and hemodynamic factors are involved in the pathogenesis of diabetic nephropathy.

Renin–angiotensin–aldosterone system (RAAS) plays an important role in pathogenesis and progression of DN. Long-standing hyperglycemia causes formation of advanced glycation end (AGE) products and activation of protein kinase C (PKC); all of which plays an important role in progression of DN.

In the presented case, the lack of response to treatment may be explained by the fact that angiotensin receptor blocker (ARB) was started at a time when proteinuria and chronic kidney disease (CKD) are already set in. And the diabetes control was not satisfactory. There is a component of AKI on CKD due to foot ulcer and cellulitis. Therefore, the patient had to undergo dialysis.

Diabetic foot is a major cause of morbidity. Macroangiopathy of blood vessels of foot are complicated by neuropathy due to uremia and diabetes mellitus. Superadded infection may aggravate the overall situation as it occurred in the presented case.

MANAGEMENT OF OTHER RISK FACTOR

Therefore, the management strategy should include optimization of glycemic control (HbA1c < 7%), control of hypertension (target BP <130/80 mm Hg), and proteinuria with angiotensin-converting enzyme inhibitor (ACEI) or ARB; aldosterone antagonist (spironolactone) and non-dihydropyridine calcium channel blocker, thiazide-like diuretic, and beta-blocker may also be added.

Cardiovascular risk reduction can be achieved by weight reduction, smoking cessation and statins, antiplatelet therapy, anemia correction by iron, erythropoiesis-stimulating agent (ESA), and blood transfusion. Patients should be educated about foot care. The best renal replacement therapy for diabetic end-stage kidney disease (ESKD) patient is living related renal transplantation (ideally preemptive transplantation). Hemodialysis is another option. Vascular access should be constructed 3–6 months before starting dialysis. Early dialysis should be planned when serum creatinine is >6 mg% and estimated glomerular filtration rate (eGFR) <15 mL/min.

Peritoneal dialysis is another option where residual renal function is better preserved with better outcome of retinopathy. Hemodynamic instability is also less in continuous ambulatory peritoneal dialysis (CAPD).

FREQUENTLY ASKED QUESTIONS

Q1. What are the conditions other than diabetic nephropathy (DN) in which we can get nodular glomerulosclerosis?

Ans.

- Membranoproliferative glomerulonephritis (MPGN)
- Amyloidosis
- Light chain deposition disease

Q2. Mention the diagnostic workup in suspected DN.

Ans.

- Estimation of urinary albumin to creatinine ratio
- Serum creatinine estimation
- eGFR
- Measurement of BP
- Fundoscopy

Q3. What are the differential diagnoses of nondiabetic renal disease in a suspected diabetic nephropathy patient?

Ans.

- Membranous glomerulonephritis (MGN)
- Focal segmental glomerulosclerosis (FSGS)
- Allergic interstitial nephritis (AIN)
- Postinfectious glomerulonephritis (PIGN)
- Immunoglobulin A nephropathy (IgAN)

Q4. What are the Indications of renal biopsy in a diabetic patient?

Ans.

- In type 1 diabetes mellitus (T1DM):
  - Absence of retinopathy inspite of proteinuria and renal impairment
  - Duration of diabetes is <5 years
  - Sudden and rapid onset of proteinuria
  - Development of nephrotic syndrome without prior microalbuminuria
- Presence of active urine sediment
- Macroscopic hematuria (glomerular origin)
- Rapid deterioration of renal function without significant proteinuria

Q5. **What percentage of diabetic retinopathy is associated with nephropathy?**

Ans.

- In type 1 diabetes mellitus (T1DM), almost 100% of retinopathy patients present with nephropathy
- In type 2 diabetes mellitus (T2DM), 50–60% nephropathy patients develop retinopathy

Q6. **What are the macrovascular complication?**

Ans. Stroke, coronary artery disease (CAD), and peripheral vascular disease (PVD).

Q7. **Which antihypertensive drugs are preferred in diabetic nephropathy?**

Ans.

- Diuretics (sodium retention and volume expansion)
- ACEI and ARB (activation of RAAS)
- Beta-blocker (activation of sympathetic nervous system)
- Target BP: Below 130/80 mm Hg

Q8. **What are the characteristic changes of diabetic retinopathy?**

Ans. Hard exudates, dot and blot hemorrhage, and neovascularization.

Note: After presenting this type of case, the examinee is usually asked to describe the detail of fundal changes, the foot ulcer and demonstration of ankle risk, vibration sense, position sense, and touch sensation.

Lupus Nephritis

■ INTRODUCTION

Mrs SK, 20 years old, Muslim, homemaker, was admitted to our hospital with the complaints of pain in multiple joints for 4 months, generalized swelling of the whole body for 2 months and fever for last 1 month. According to the patient's statement, she was reasonably well about 4 months back, then she noticed pain in multiple joints which was insidious in onset and involving small and large joints of upper and lower limbs, predominantly upper limbs, moderate in intensity, symmetrical, inflammatory in nature with morning stiffness >1 hour, not relieved by rest but reduced by pain killers. She also complained of excessive hair fall and multiple painless oral ulcers for same duration. Then she developed swelling all over the body 2 months back, initially appeared in face, then gradually involved rest of the body. The swelling was associated with breathlessness, cough, and productive sputum, which was white and frothy, no hemoptysis was noted. She has no history of reduction in urine output, no history of passage of dark-colored urine, but patient mentioned about passing of frothy urine. She had no history of chest pain, paroxysmal nocturnal dyspnea, and orthopnea. In addition to that she complained of fever for last 1 month which was continued in nature, not associated with chills and rigor, relieved partially by antipyretics, highest recorded temperature was 102°F. With these complaints, she was admitted in our hospital and during hospital stay on, she developed generalized tonic-clonic seizure which persisted for 5 minutes, associated with visual aura, headache, and postictal confusion. There was no history of tongue bite or urinary or fecal incontinence. She was managed with intramuscular (IM) diazepam and intravenous (IV) phenytoin. There was no history of previous seizure prior to this episode.

This lady has no significant history of past illness. She is nonsmoker, nonalcoholic, she has no history of contact with any tuberculosis patient. She has one son who is in good health. Her parents are alive and well. Her all other family members are healthy. She comes from a middle class family, her husband works at a textile industry, earning 20,000 per month. They live in tin-shed house and drink tube well water. She is immunized according to Expanded Programme on Immunization (EPI) schedule. Pneumococcal and influenza vaccine was given during the hospital course. She is a normally menstruating woman. She has no history of abortion.

On examination, her appearance was ill-looking, puffy face, she was mildly anemic, her pulse was 76 bpm, her blood pressure (BP) was 140/80 mm Hg, temperature 99°F, moderately edematous, painless oral ulcers present and bedside urine dipstick showed +++ proteinuria. Jaundice, cyanosis, clubbing, koilonychias, leukonychia, and lymphadenopathy. Mild tenderness present in the small joint of hands, wrist, elbow, and knee joint. There was no swelling of joints and no deformity.

Respiratory and cardiovascular system examination revealed no abnormality. Fundoscopy is normal.

INVESTIGATIONS

Urine R/M/E showed albumin +++, red blood cell (RBC): 8–10/high power field (HPF), white blood cell (WBC): 6–10/HFP, cast: granular 4–8/HPF, 24 hours urinary total protein: 4.02 g/day, hemoglobin: 10.1 g/dL, erythrocyte sedimentation rate (ESR) (in 1st hour) 105 mm, WBC count: 9,000, N—88%, L—11%, platelet count: 270,000, serum albumin: 21 g/L, serum creatinine: 1.45 mg/dL, serum electrolytes: Na—130 mmol/L, K—4.4 mmol/L, Cl—103.8 mmol/L, TCO_2—27.1 mmol/L, serum calcium: 1.7 mmol/L corrected Ca (1.2 mmol/L), serum iron: 13 mcg/dL (normal range: 60–170 mcg/dL), serum ferritin: 716 ng/mL (normal range: 24–336 ng/mL), total iron-binding capacity (TIBC) 194 mcg/dL (normal range: 240–450 mcg/dL), transferrin saturation (TSAT): 6.70%, anti-hepatitis C virus (HCV), HBsAg, anti-HBc: negative, prothrombin time: control 12.00 seconds patient 30 seconds, international normalized ratio (INR): 1.13, activated partial thromboplastin time (APTT): Control 26 seconds patient 30 seconds, bleeding time (BT): 3 minutes, clotting time (CT): 6 minutes, echocardiography showed: Moderate pericardial effusion (14 mm), and ejection fraction (EF)—58%.

Ultrasonography of Whole Abdomen
- Both kidneys are normal in size, shape, and position.
- Normal corticomedullary differentiation
- Moderate ascites present

Noncontrast Computed Tomography Scan of Chest

- Inflammatory lesion with subsegmental consolidation in right lung, more marked in middle and lower lobes
- Right-sided mild pleural effusion and mild pericardial effusion

Magnetic Resonance Imaging of Brain

- Acute infarcts **(Fig. 1)**

Renal Biopsy

Light microscopic examination **(Figs. 2A to D)**:
- *Glomerulus*: Number-18, size-enlarged, cellularity-proliferation of endocapillary cells, matrix-increased (++), glomerular basement membrane (GBM)—thick
- *Tubules*: Tubular atrophy—mild, epithelium-features of protein reabsorption, tubular basement membrane (TBM), thick in atrophic tubules, cast—hyaline, RBC, and granular
- *Interstitium*: Inflammation—chronic, mild

Direct immune fluorescence finding:
- Immunoglobulin G (IgG)—GBM, mesangial deposition, granular, and intensity is (++++)
- IgA—GBM, mesangial deposition, granular, and intensity is (+)
- C3—GBM, mesangial deposition, granular, and intensity is (++)
- C1q—GBM, mesangial deposition, granular, and intensity is (++)
- Kappa—GBM, mesangial deposition, granular, and intensity is (++)
- Lamda—GBM, mesangial deposition, granular, and intensity is (++)

Comment: Diffuse proliferative lupus nephritis (LN) (class IV)

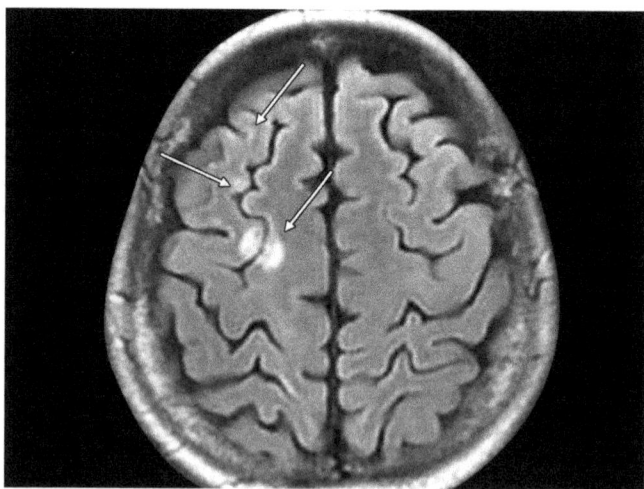

FIG. 1: Magnetic resonance imaging (MRI) of brain showing infarct (arrows).

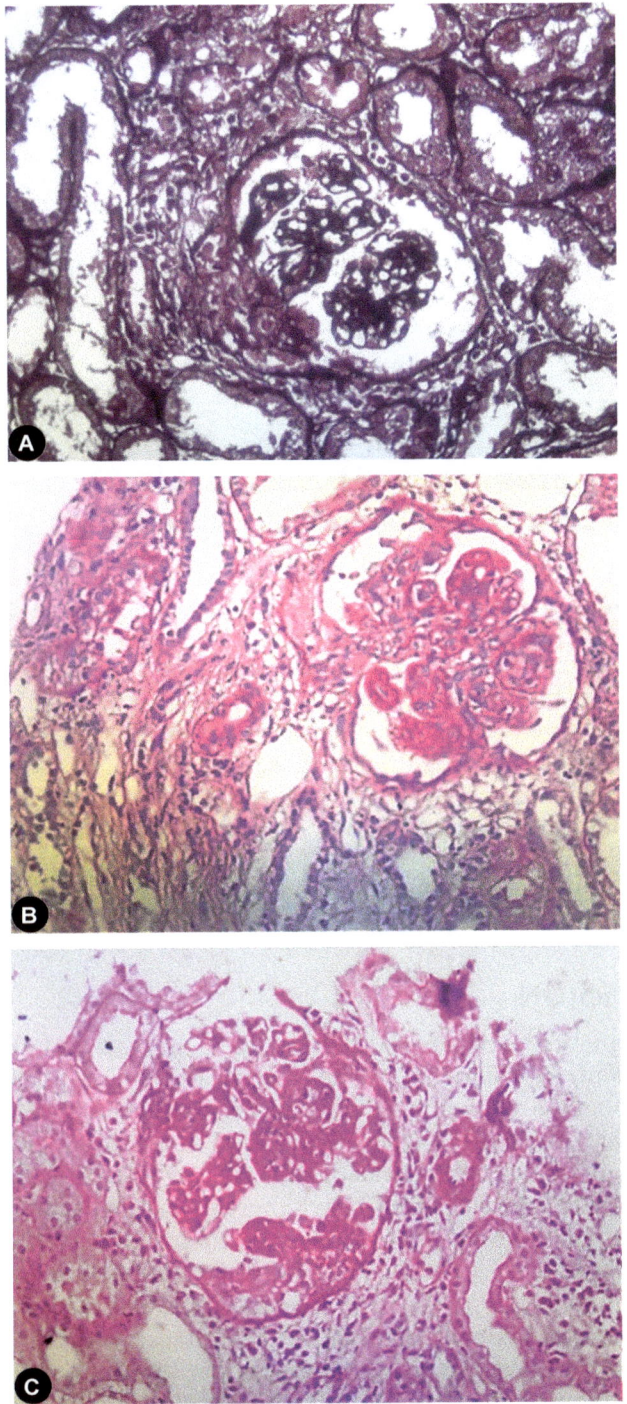

FIGS. 2A TO D: *Continued*

Continued

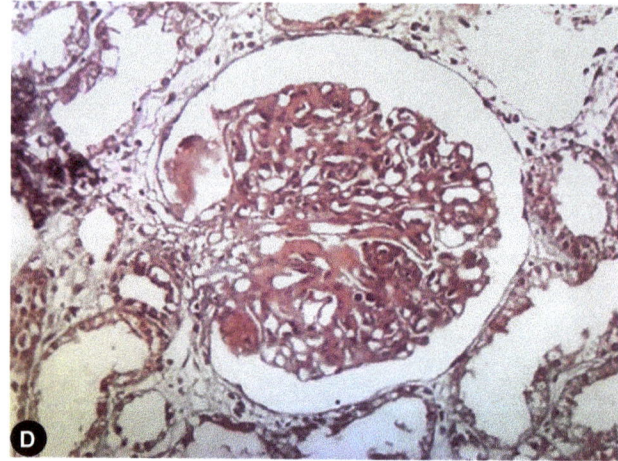

FIGS. 2A TO D: Lupus nephritis class IV (histopathology slides).

■ TREATMENT

The patient got several medications after admission in our hospital. Those were: Injection methylprednisolone 1 g IV daily for 3 days followed oral prednisolone 1 mg/kg/day. Injection lasix (20 mg)—1 amp IV 12 hourly, injection phenytoin 750 mg diluted in 200 mL normal saline @30 d/min, followed by injection phenytoin (150 mg)—1 amp IM tds for 7 days, tablet levetiracetam 250 mg bd, tablet paracetamol (500)—per oral (po) sos, after renal biopsy, she was given treatment according to KDIGO guidelines for class 4 LN with IV cyclophosphamide 750 mg/m^2 1st dose and was advised to follow-up for further treatment.

■ DISCUSSION

Systemic lupus erythematosus (SLE) can affect any organ of the body. But renal and neurological involvement is prognostically bad. Although SLE is female preponderant disease, LN affects both gender equally. However, it is more severe in men and children. Renal involvement occurs in about 60% adult lupus patients. Some patients may present with renal involvement (membranous LN) at the beginning without other systemic features. Renal involvement is characterized by active urinary sediment proteinuria (hematuria and RBC cast) and hypertension. Some other glomerular diseases mimic SLE. These are Henoch–Schönlein purpura nephritis (immunoglobulin A deposition in HSP and full house deposition in SLE).

Pauci immune rapidly progressive glomerulonephritis (RPGN) with positive antineutrophil cytoplasmic antibody (ANCA) may be confused with LN (serology and renal biopsy). Patients positive for both ANCA and antinuclear antibody (ANA) or anti-ds DNA but having no immune deposits on renal biopsy be treated as pauci immune glomerulonephritis (GN).

Antineutrophil cytoplasmic antibody positivity has got no significance in an established case of SLE. Bacterial endocarditis and cryoglobulinemia can also mimic SLE.

Neurological involvement usually presents with headache, psychosis, seizure, and coma.

Patients with severe proliferative LN and patients with neurological involvement need aggressive treatment as has been done in the present case. In most cases, acute renal condition improves in 3 months of treatment and by 6 months almost all responding patients show improvement in glomerular filtration rate (GFR), decline in proteinuria and serologic markers such as anti-ds DNA antibody titers and complement levels also improve during this time period.

Relapse rate varies from 35 to 60%. Elevation of anti-ds DNA antibody titer and decrease in complement level may herald a relapse. Monitoring during remission includes BP measurement, estimation of GFR, proteinuria, and urinary sediment.

To stop treatment is often possible after 5 years or more when there is no proteinuria, normal serological tests, and stable renal function.

FREQUENTLY ASKED QUESTIONS

Q1. What is SLICC criteria for diagnosis of LN?

Ans. SLICC criteria require at 4 of 17 criteria including 1 of the 11 clinical criteria and 1 of 6 immunologic criteria or that the patient has biopsy-proven nephritis compatible with SLE in the presence of ANA or anti-ds DNA positivity.

Q2. What are the types of flares in LN?

Ans. Two types of flares:
1. *Proteinuria flare*: An isolated increase in proteinuria typically at least doubling and above 1 g/24 hours
2. *Nephritic flare*: Appearance of glomerular hematuria or red cell casts with proteinuria, with or without hypertension and a decline in GFR

Q3. What are the indications of repeat renal biopsy?

Ans.
- At the time of flare
- Rapidly declining GFR
- To detect class transformation and activity and chronicity index

Q4. Treatment of class IV lupus.

Ans. *Induction*: Injection methylprednisolone 1 g IV daily for 3 days or oral prednisolone 1 mg/kg/day

Plus

Oral mycophenolate mofetil (MMF) 1.0–1.5 g bid for 6 months

Or

Replace MMF with IV cyclophosphamide

Or

Replace MMF with oral cyclophosphamide 1–3 mg/kg/day for 3–6 months

Maintenance:

Low-dose prednisolone 5–10 mg/day or alternate day plus oral MMF 0.5–1 g bid

Or

Replace MMF with oral azathioprine 1–2 mg/kg/day

Q5.   What is Eurolupus regimen?

Ans. Cyclophosphamide 500 mg IV every 2 weeks for six doses (total dose 3 g), then switching to azathioprine maintenance therapy (2 mg/kg/day). Less toxicity and less infection complication.

Q6.   Treatment of type V c/d.

Ans. Treatment is same as class IV.

Q7.   Transplantation in lupus patients.

Ans.

- Wait until 6–12 months on dialysis (lupus is not active).
- Many patients have burnt out disease by the time they reach end-stage renal disease (ESRD).
- Some patients rapidly develop irreversible renal failure and needs renal replacement therapy as well as aggressive treatment for active disease, but need to wait for 6–12 months before transplantation.
- Some patients with antiphospholipid syndrome require anticoagulation to prevent arteriovenous fistula or graft clotting.
- Cross matching of donors with lupus patients may be difficult because the sera may contain antilymphocyte antibody (false positive cross match).

Q8.   What is the background drug in the treatment of LN?

Ans. Hydroxychloroquine.

Q9.   What is remission in LN?

Ans. Reduction in proteinuria below 0.5 g/24 hours or urine protein creatinine ratio below 0.5 mg/mmol, absence of glomerular hematuria or red cell casts and normalization or stabilization of GFR.

Antineutrophil Cytoplasmic Antibody-positive Glomerulonephritis

INTRODUCTION

A 51-year-old diabetic female presented with bilateral leg swelling and dry cough for 1 year; she was diabetic for 10 years. She was reasonably well 1 year ago, then she noticed occasional swelling of legs and with treatment, her symptoms resolved partially. Then, she developed dry cough, more after waking up in the morning, not associated with fever or breathlessness, not aggravated by cold or dust exposure but progressively deteriorating. On evaluation, she had high erythrocyte sedimentation rate (ESR) and lung lesions in the form of multiple-rounded opacities in both lungs. Tuberculin test was negative.

Then, computed tomography (CT)-guided fine-needle aspiration cytology (FNAC) from right lung lesion was done which was compatible with granulomatous inflammation. She was put on antituberculosis (TB) drugs empirically but after about 4 weeks, her general condition deteriorated and anti-TB drugs were stopped. CT-guided FNAC from right lung lesion was done again which was suggestive of moderate interstitial fibrosis and inflammation, no obvious malignancy. Then, positron emission tomography (PET)-CT scan was done which revealed bilateral metabolically active chronic granulomatous lung lesion. Then, pulmonary lobectomy of right middle lobe was done and histopathology report suggested necrotizing granulomatous lesion. Meanwhile, she developed increased swelling of legs and noticed frothy urine. Then, she was referred to nephrologist for proteinuria workup and after evaluation, her 24-hour urinary total protein (UTP) was found to be 5.4 g. And vasculitis panel showed positive cytoplasmic antineutrophil cytoplasmic antibody (c-ANCA). She is diabetic patient for 11 years and was on oral hypoglycemic drug with good control. She has occasional shortness of breath on exertion but no orthopnea or paroxysmal nocturnal dyspnea, had mechanical right knee joint pain, weight loss of about 5 kg in 6 months.

She has no history of skin rash, oral ulcer and photosensitivity, redness of eye, sinusitis, or rhinitis. She has hypopigmented skin change from 5 years of age. She has history of cholecystectomy, hysterectomy, and herniotomy. She is treated with olmesartan, montelukast, diuretics, etc.

On examination, she is mildly anemic, had bilateral pedal edema, multiple hypopigmented skin lesion involving different area of body with intact sensation. Fundoscopy is normal. There is no signs of diabetic neuropathy. Examination of chest revealed features of right-sided pleural effusion/pleural thickening/mass lesion.

Bedside urine examination shows protein +++.

INVESTIGATIONS

Urine R/M/E: Protein +++, red blood cell (RBC): nil, pus cells: 6–8, cast: nil, urine C/S: no growth 24 hours urinary total protein was 5.4 g, serum albumin: 18.4 g/L, serum creatinine: 0.8 mg/dL, electrolytes normal, antinuclear antibody (ANA), and anti-ds DNA antibody were negative. Complements C3 and C4 are normal. Serum angiotensin-converting enzyme (ACE) 57 U/L and 24 hours urine 5HIAA is low, c-ANCA is positive (8.3 U/mL), perinuclear antineutrophil cytoplasmic antibodies (p-ANCA) is negative (4.2 U/mL); anti-PR3 is positive (25.3 IU/mL). Ultrasonography showed: Both kidneys are enlarged and echogenic, mild hepatomegaly, and right-sided pleural effusion. Renal biopsy revealed necrotizing vasculitis **(Figs. 1 and 2)**.

Chest X-ray posteroanterior (P/A) view: Multiple well-defined almost rounded opacities are noted at both upper and lower zones and part of right mid zone. Rest of lung fields are clear and right-sided minimal pleural effusion **(Fig. 3)**.

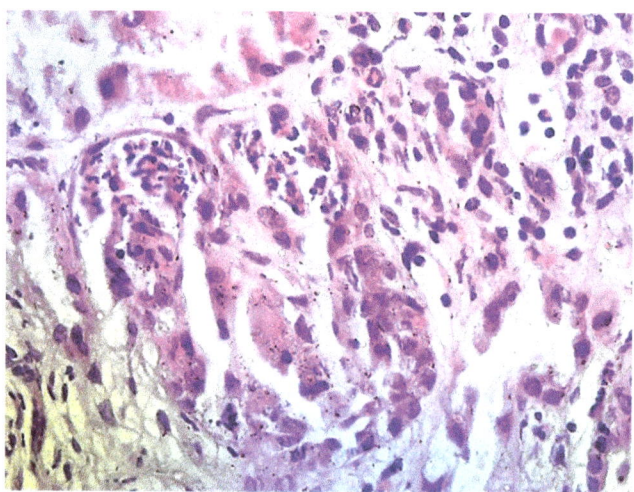

FIG. 1: Hematoxylin and Eosin 40× (necrotic segment).

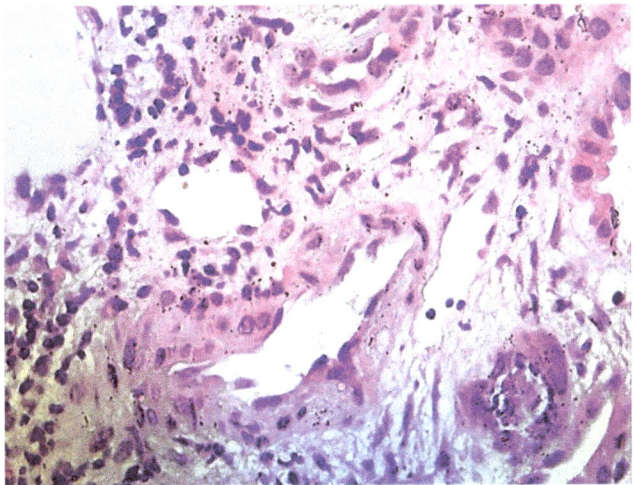

FIG. 2: Hematoxylin and Eosin 40× vessel wall inflammation.

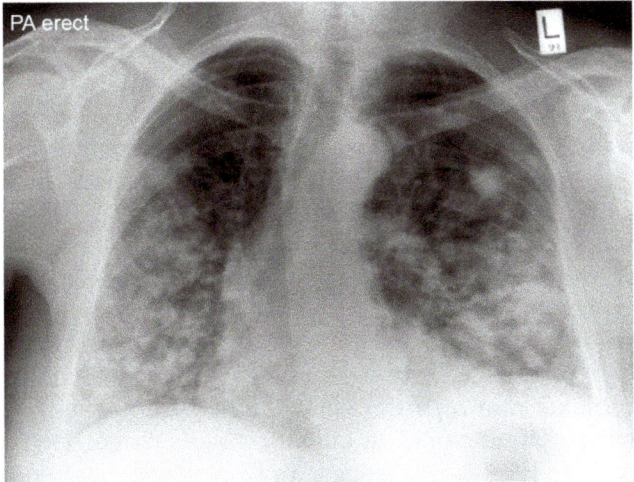

FIG. 3: The chest radiograph showed multiple pulmonary nodules with the presence of air bronchograms particularly in the lower zones with no cavitation or lobar collapse.

She was diagnosed as a case of granulomatosis with polyangiitis (GPA). She was treated with intravenous methylprednisolone 1 g IV daily for 3 days along with IV cyclophosphamide 0.5–1 g/m^2 body surface area. The methylprednisolone was followed by oral prednisolone 1 mg/kg/day.

■ DISCUSSION

Granulomatosis with polyangiitis, previously known as Wegener's granulomatosis, is a granulomatous disease involving upper and lower respiratory tract. Necrotizing vasculitis involves small- and medium-sized blood vessels including necrotizing glomerulonephritis. ARA criteria for diagnosis includes: Nephritic urinary sediment, abnormal chest finding, nasal or oral inflammation, and granulomatous lesion on biopsy.

The common manifestations of GPA include cough (34%), hemoptysis (18%), nasal congestion and epistaxis (11%), pulmonary infiltrate (71%), purpuric rash (13%), and renal impairment (11%).

The patient under discussion presented with occasional swelling of legs (renal involvement), urine examination showed nephrotic range proteinuria but no active sediment and cough (respiratory tract involvement). Her chest X-ray showed multiple-rounded opacities. Repeated biopsy from lung lesion revealed granulomatous lesion, which was considered as of tubercular origin and antituberculosis drugs given for 1 month with no improvement. Repeat CT-guided biopsy revealed interstitial inflammation and fibrosis and PET-CT suggested metabolically active granulomatous lung lesion. Then, pulmonary lobectomy (right middle lube) was done and histopathologists (of different centers) were divided on their opinion, one opinion was "necrotizing sarcoid granuloma" and the other opinion was "inflammatory myofibroblastic tumor."

Our patient did not present with typical respiratory symptoms. Only respiratory symptom was cough. Radiologically, there was pulmonary infiltrate. But biopsy of pulmonary lesion showed granulomatous lesion. Differential diagnoses were TB, sarcoidosis, carcinoid tumor, etc.

Renal manifestations include nephrotic range proteinuria without active urine sediment and raised serum creatinine. As the patient was diabetic, the proteinuria might also be due to diabetic nephropathy. But here diabetic retinopathy and neuropathy were absent. When c-ANCA directed against PR3 became positive (very specific for GPA) and renal biopsy revealed necrotizing vasculitis; then, the diagnosis of GPA became obvious.

The combination of high-dose glucocorticoid and cyclophosphamide is the mainstay of treatment. Our patient was given injection methylprednisolone 1 g IV daily for 3 days along with IV cyclophosphamide 0.5–1 g/m^2 body surface area. The methylprednisolone is followed by oral prednisolone 1 mg/kg/day tapering to alternate day regimen after 1 week depending on response and discontinued in 3–4 months.

Intravenous cyclophosphamide is given at nine repeat cycles, first three cycles at 2 weeks' intervals and the rest six cycles at 3 weeks' interval.

Our patient improved with this regimen. Cyclophosphamide may also be given orally 2 mg/kg/day for 3 months.

Rituximab may also be used in case of refractory disease and in patients where cyclophosphamide is contraindicated. Rituximab may be used as induction agent as well as for maintenance therapy.

For maintenance therapy, cyclophosphamide may be converted to azathioprine after 3–6 months. Plasma exchange could be considered for patients requiring dialysis or with rapidly increasing serum creatinine and in patients with diffuse alveolar hemorrhage, in patients with overlap syndrome of antineutrophil cytoplasmic antibody (ANCA) vasculitis and antiglomerular basement membrane (GBM) disease.

FREQUENTLY ASKED QUESTIONS

Q1. When rituximab is preferred?

Ans.

- Children and adolescent
- Premenopausal women
- Men concerned about fertility
- Relapsing disease
- PR3 ANCA disease

Q2. How a relapse is diagnosed?

Ans. Relapse is diagnosed on the basis of clinical and pathological evidence of recurrence of disease; not only by an increase in ANCA titer alone.

Q3. What is the treatment of relapse?

Ans. Reinstitution of treatment similar to the induction protocol is mostly practiced. A number of drugs like cyclophosphamide, rituximab, IVIG, and MMF in combination with methotrexate or azathioprine.

Q4. How do you plan transplantation in ANCA-associated vasculitis (AAV)?

Ans. Transplantation may be delayed until patients are in complete clinical remission for at least 6 months. Persistence of ANCA positivity should not delay transplantation.

Post-transplant Thrombotic Microangiopathy

▌ INTRODUCTION

A 36-year-old male, known case of chronic kidney disease (CKD) stage 5 on maintenance hemodialysis with difficult to control hypertension, underwent living related donor transplantation. His primary renal disease was unknown. Donor was his mother with one haplotype match. Post-transplant immunosuppression consisted of intravenous (IV) methylprednisolone 500 mg/day for 3 days followed by oral prednisolone 1 mg/kg/day, mycophenolate mofetil 1 g/day, and cyclosporine 8 mg/kg/day in two divided doses.

In the immediate postoperative period, urine output increased till the third postoperative day and then urine output started to decrease and became nil out put on the fifth postoperative day. Patient became anemic and her blood pressure was increased to 160/95 mm Hg. Her serum creatinine was 7 mg%, serum sodium 135 mmol/L, serum potassium 5.9 mmol/L, serum chloride 117 mmol/L, uric acid 9.2 mg, peripheral blood film showed dimorphic anemia with microcytes and macrocytes, with elongated cells, polychromatic cells, few schistocytes, and crenated cells. Reticulocyte count was 1.42%, serum bilirubin: Total 0.5 mg/dL, indirect—0.3 mg/dL, direct—0.2 mg/dL, fibrin degradation product (FDP): 8.9 mg/L, D-dimer: 1.94 µg/mL, Coombs test: direct—negative, indirect—negative. Cytomegalovirus (CMV) and BK virus DNA were negative. A clinical diagnosis of acute rejection/acute tubular necrosis was made. Renal biopsy was done. In the meantime, IV methylprednisolone 1 g IV daily started and the patient was put on alternate day hemodialysis, three units of blood transfusion was given using leukocyte filter.

Renal biopsy report became available showing fibrinoid necrosis and platelet fibrin thrombi in capillaries and arterioles at the glomerular vascular pole and vacuolization of proximal tubular epithelial cell cytoplasm. Due to lack of facility, C4d staining could not be done. A diagnosis of post-transplant calcineurin inhibitor (CNI) induced thrombotic microangiopathy was made. Cyclosporine was switched to everolimus. Five sessions of therapeutic plasma exchange were done. His renal function improved, hemoglobin and platelet count improved. He was discharged with serum creatinine 2.2 mg%, hemoglobin (Hb) 9.2 g/dL, and platelet count 180,000/m^2.

▋ DISCUSSION

Thrombotic microangiopathy (TMA) denotes noninflammatory small vessel vasculopathies which result from severe endothelial cell injury/necrosis that culminates in variable degree of organ ischemia. The pathological diagnosis of TMA requires the presence of one or more of the following:

- Microvascular thrombi
- A glomerular capillary occlusion which results from subendothelial deposits of the electron lucent material
- A severe subendothelial widening

Thrombotic microangiopathy is relatively more common in transplant patients than in the general population, presumably due to the clustering of the risk factors. Post-transplant thrombotic microangiopathy (PT-TMA) can be "recurrent," occurring in patient with a previous history of hemolytic uremic syndrome (HUS)/thrombotic thrombocytopenic purpura (TTP) or it may be "de-novo," occurring for the first time post-transplantation. The USRDS data analysis quoted the incidence of "de-novo" TMA as 0.8%; however, various studies have reported its incidence to range from 4 to 14%. This condition can be triggered by renal ischemia, antibody-mediated rejection (AMR), malignancy, viral infections [CMV, influenza A, parvovirus B19, BK polyomavirus, human immunodeficiency virus (HIV), and human herpesvirus 6 (HHV-6)], antiphospholipid antibodies, anticardiolipin antibodies in hepatitis C virus (HCV)-positive patients and drugs (CNI, antiviral agents), and can occur in patients who are on CNIs, affecting 3–14% of the patients who are on cyclosporine and approximately 1% of the patients who are on tacrolimus. The precise mechanism of CNI-induced TMA is not clear; however, it is attributed to the vasoconstriction, endothelial toxicity, and prothrombotic and antifibrinolytic effects of the drug. The trough levels of cyclosporine are not predictive of developing TMA and the rising serum creatinine levels may be the only alteration reflecting renal dysfunction.

The clinical presentation may be variable. Some patients present with "localized" TMA manifested by only worsening of renal function and others present with features of "systemic" TMA which is characterized by microangiopathic hemolysis and thrombocytopenia.

The patients with the localized CNI-induced TMA often respond to the reduction, temporary discontinuation, or the conversion of CNI, usually without a plasma exchange, unlike AMR-induced TMA which requires one or more alternative like a plasma exchange, an intravenous immunoglobulin, and the anti-CD20 antibody. Thus, differentiating these two entities which have entirely different pathogeneses and outcomes is of utmost importance. A distinction is not possible on the basis of the morphology alone. The peritubular capillary C4d positivity is present in AMR and it is a useful discriminator; however, the absence of a C4d staining does not exclude AMR, as 10% of the cases are C4d negative. These cases require additional serological studies [anti-human leukocyte antigen (HLA)-donor antibodies] and a meticulous clinic pathological correlation. An irregular intimal proliferation with a subendothelial neutrophilic and mononuclear infiltration, peritubular capillaritis, and an arterial fibrinoid necrosis, with a general involvement of the entire vascular tree, are the features of AMR, whereas the fibrin thrombi which focally affect the arterioles at the glomerular vascular poles and distally extend into the glomerular capillaries in a segmental fashion, suggest CNI-induced TMA.

The type of TMA in our case is de novo type. And the clinical manifestation is systemic. Therefore, an improved renal function was seen following the withdrawal of cyclosporine and institution of plasma exchange.

FREQUENTLY ASKED QUESTIONS

Q1. What is TMA?

Ans. Thrombotic microangiopathy is an acute syndrome characterized by microangiopathic hemolytic anemia, thrombocytopenia, and variable signs of organ injury due to platelet thrombosis in microcirculation.

Q2. What are the differential diagnoses of TMA?

Ans. In case of thrombocytopenia, microangiopathic hemolytic anemia, and acute kidney injury (AKI)—the differential diagnoses are: Hypertensive emergency, disseminated intravascular coagulation (DIC), and endemic hanta virus infection.

Q3. What are the major clinical types of TMA?

Ans.

- HUS
- TTP

Q4. What is the treatment of post-transplant HUS?

Ans.

- Symptomatic
- Removal of inciting factor

  Drug withdrawal or dose reduction and plasma therapy have got high success rate (84%); in case of de novo cyclosporine and tacrolimus-associated condition. Intravenous immunoglobulin G (IgG) infusion may also be given once remission is achieved; possible immunosuppressive treatments may include a decreased dose of cyclosporine or tacrolimus, change from cyclosporine to tacrolimus or vice versa, and avoidance of CNI and use of mycophenolate mofetil or everolimus.

Transplantation in a Patient with Lower Urinary Tract Abnormality

◼ INTRODUCTION

Mr HA, a 32-year-old male, was diagnosed as a case of bilateral hydroureteronephrosis due to posterior urethral valve and had a transurethral fulguration. Since then, he has been suffering from purulent discharge during micturition. Later on, left-sided ureteroneocystostomy was done for vesicoureteric reflux. A couple of years later, he visited another center where he was diagnosed as detrusor sphincter dyssynergia with bilateral hydroureteronephrosis with chronic kidney disease (CKD) stage V and hypertension. After about 5 years, he had to undergo left-sided nephrectomy for pyonephrosis and histopathology of the kidney revealed chronic pyelonephritis. Nephrectomy was followed by several episodes of urinary tract infection (UTI). Later on, urodynamic study and cystoscopy were done which revealed bladder neck hypertrophy for which modified bladder neck incision (BNI) was given. Later on, laparoscopic right-sided nephrectomy was carried out due to persistent UTI and histopathology of which also revealed chronic pyelonephritis. Then, he was put on maintenance hemodialysis. He received several units of whole blood transfusion during his course of illness.

Finally, he underwent kidney transplantation for end-stage renal failure secondary to obstructive nephropathy and chronic pyelonephritis. He received kidney from his 52-year-old hypertensive mother. Her echocardiogram was normal, she had no proteinuria and no retinopathy. Both T cells and B cells cross-match and auto cross-match was negative at 5°C, RT and 37°C, and with dithiothreitol (DTT). Immunosuppression was provided based on the transplant center's current standard of care, induction was given with methylprednisolone (Solumedrol) 1 g per operatively and 500 mg for the next 2 days following which he was put on maintenance therapy comprised of cyclosporine 8 mg/kg/day in two divided doses, mycophenolate mofetil 750 mg twice daily and oral prednisolone 0.5 mg/kg/day and which was subsequently tapered. Induction with basiliximab was not given. The patient was cytomegalovirus seropositive (IgG positive) and so was the donor. Antiviral prophylaxis consisted of valganciclovir. Warm ischemic time was 1 minutes and 54 seconds. Cold ischemic time was 22 minutes. Total surgery was uneventful except the control of blood pressure (BP) of recipient. Urine came out immediately after anastomosis of the renal artery.

On the day of operation, his BP was 220/120 mm Hg because of which he was shifted to transplant intensive care unit, where he was put on IV glyceryl trinitrate (GTN) infusion at the rate of 0.3 mg/h and it was gradually up titrated to 3 mg/h. Despite all these measures, his BP remained 200/100 mm Hg. So, the day after surgery, he was put on infusion labetalol 15 mg/min and a maximum of 200 mg was given. Then, his BP dropped to about 160–170/90–110 mm Hg. So, oral antihypertensive nifedipine and prazosin were also added. His urine output which was initially 2.3 L/day then kept decreasing and came down to 150 mL/day but onward, it further dropped down to only about 50 mL/day and finally became nil. Hemodialysis was started from 8th postoperative day and since then he was on intermittent hemodialysis. Physical examination revealed facial puffiness, mild anemia, and mild edema. Pulse 88 bpm, BP: 200/120 mm Hg, temperature: 99°F, weight: 68 kg, functioning arteriovenous (AV) fistula on left forearm.

Abdominal examination revealed multiple scars in right and left lumbar, right hypochondriac and umbilical region, the longest one extending from right iliac fossa to the public symphysis. On palpation, there was a bean-shaped mass situated in the right iliac fossa. It measured about 10 cm × 6 cm, was mildly tender having rounded margin. Shifting dullness was detected on percussion. No bruit could be heard over the mass.

All other systemic examinations including nervous system, cardiovascular system, and respiratory system were unremarkable.

During the immediate postoperative period (Tables 1 to 3), he had a good diuresis but it became only 2.3 L/day on the 1st postoperative day and decreased to 1.5 L/day on the 2nd and 785 mL/day on the 3rd postoperative day. At that time his BP was 150/100 mm Hg. His serum creatinine fell to 3.4 mg/dL on 1st postoperative day but rose to 4.16 mg/dL on 2nd postoperative day warranting urgent duplex study of both renal vessels on 2nd postoperative day to reveal <50% stenosis in the absence of any thrombus at the renal artery anastomotic site and normal intrarenal arterial flow with mild perinephric collection. Injection methylprednisolone was continued for another couple of days. But as his serum creatinine was not decreasing, an allograft biopsy was done on 12th postoperative day with a diagnosis of acute tubular necrosis (ATN). Acute rejection could not be ruled out. Despite this, plasma exchange was planned but was again not possible due to financial constraint of the patient. Besides, there were no features of CNI toxicity and cyclosporine C_2 level was within normal range. His serum creatinine never became

TABLE 1: Blood pressure (BP), urine output, and some laboratory parameters.

	Pretransplant	Day of surgery	1st POD	2nd POD	3rd POD	4th POD	5th POD	6th POD	7th POD	8th POD	9th POD	10th POD
BP (mm Hg)	180/100	220/130	200/110	150/100	160/100	150/90	140/90	160/100	150/90	150/100	170/90	
Urine output	Nil	10 L	2.3 L	1.5 L	785 mL	7,000 mL	345 mL	270 mL	170 mL	170 mL	90 mL	100 mL
Serum creatinine (mg/dL)	5.8	6.4	3.4	4.16	5.53	6.2	7.1	7.3 Neo	7.2 HD	5.2 Tacro	6.1	6.2
Serum electrolyte (mmol/L)	139 4.1	139 3.9	131 4.4	128 4.4		125 4.9		129 3.9	131 3.5	134 3.2		133 3.1
Hb (g/dL) TC/Neutrophil	9.5 4,100	7.8 7,000	7.3 14,000	6.8 15,000 92%		7.4 12,300 90%		8.6 6,900 87%	8.8 11,300 79%			9.4 107,00 85%
RBS (mmol/L)	6.9		7.2			4.6			4.6			5.7

(POD: postoperative day)

TABLE 2: Follow up continuation.							
	14th POD	16th POD	19th POD	23rd POD	25th POD	27th POD	28th POD
Urine output	40 mL	20 mL	10 mL	20 mL	10 mL	10 mL	10 mL
Serum creatinine (mg/dL)	5.29	5.5	6.5	5.6	5.3		5.4
Hb (g/dL)	9	9	9	7.9	6.9		
TC	15,500	14,600	12,500	8,600	8,000		
RBS (mmol/L)	6	5.3			4.6		6.4

(POD: postoperative day)

TABLE 3: Urine R/M/E and C/S.			
	Pre-transplant	4th POD	8th POD
Protein	++++	+++	+++
Sugar	Nil	Nil	Nil
Pus cell/HPF	Plenty	40–50	Plenty
RBC/HPF	20–30	Plenty	Plenty
C/S	Pseudomonas ($>10^5$/cfu)	No growth	Pseudomonas ($>10^5$/cfu)

(RBC: red blood cell; POD: postoperative day)

normal after renal transplantation rather it kept progressively rising. Hemodialysis was started on 8th postoperative day due to progressive rise in his serum creatinine and features of volume overload and he was put on intermittent hemodialysis since then. His hemoglobin was within 8–9 g/dL. Serum electrolyte and blood sugar were within normal limit, although there was hyponatremia immediately after surgery; possibly due to dilutional effect. He received several courses of antibiotics according to sensitivity report due to persistent post-transplant UTI. But the patient was afebrile and there were no systemic symptoms. Liver function tests were within reference limits. His chest X-ray posteroinferior (PA) view showed minimal left-sided pleural effusion. Blood biochemistry showed hypocalcemia. Duplex study of both renal vessels was repeated on 23rd postoperative day and showed increased resistance at intrarenal arterial flow with no detectable thrombus in renal vein but <50% stenosis at renal artery anastomotic site.

DISCUSSION

Familiarity with management of patients with abnormal lower urinary tract is important because such patients are about 20–30% of renal transplant recipients. Correction of structural abnormalities and optimizing storage and emptying function of bladder is recommended. Abnormal bladders must be assessed urodynamically before and after surgery.

Our patient had posterior urethral valve and reflux nephropathy. He underwent fulguration and left-sided ureteroneocystostomy. Even after undergoing these surgical procedures, he developed chronic pyelonephritis and CKD stage V.

He was evaluated thoroughly as a prospective recipient. His mother came forward to donate one of her kidneys to the son. She was hypertensive (marginal donor) but she had no features of end-organ involvement from hypertension [no proteinuria, no left ventricular hypertrophy (LVH) on echocardiography, and no evidence of hypertensive retinopathy].

The patient had a good diuresis immediately after transplantation but gradually the urine output was decreased and BP and serum creatinine were raised. Renal biopsy was inconclusive. This could be a case of acute antibody-mediated rejection which could not be established due to unavailability of C4d staining and donor specific antibody (DSA) test.

Finally, there was irreversible graft loss and patient was back on maintenance hemodialysis.

FREQUENTLY ASKED QUESTIONS

Q1. What is a marginal living donor?

Ans. A marginal donor is one who is ≥70 years of age, one who is <60 years of age with several risk factors, or a donor who is 60–69 years of age with at least one of the following risk factors: Severe hypertension, diabetes mellitus, or significant cardiovascular disease.

Q2. What is a marginal cadaveric kidney donor?

Ans.

- Age >60 years
- Age >50 years but with any of the following:
  - Hypertension
  - Cerebrovascular cause of brain death
  - Preretrieval serum creatinine level >1.5 mg% with a degree of glomerulosclerosis >15%

Q3. Is lower tract obstruction a contraindication of renal transplantation?

Ans. When renal failure results from underlying urological anomalies, e.g., posterior urethral valve, neurogenic bladder, etc., it is assumed that the abnormal bladder that contributed to the destruction of the native kidneys might adversely influence the outcome of the transplanted kidney. Correction of structural anomalies and optimization of storage and emptying functions of the bladder are often recommended before transplantation.

Therefore, abnormal bladder must be assessed urodynamically before and after transplantation.

Preemptive Renal Transplantation

■ INTRODUCTION

Mr M, 48 years of age, a known case of hypertension (HTN) for 11 years, chronic kidney disease (CKD) for 8 years, and newly diagnosed diabetes mellitus (DM) for 2 months, came to Bangabandhu Sheikh Mujib Medical University (BSMMU) hospital for renal transplantation. Patient was apparently well 11 years back, then he was diagnosed as HTN incidentally. Since then he is on antihypertensive drug regularly. After 2 years, he consulted with a medicine specialist for uncontrolled HTN and anxiety disorder. After evaluation, he was diagnosed as having renal impairment with serum creatinine 2.3 mg/dL. During last 8 years, he visited many nephrologists and treated conservatively. During this period, his serum creatinine was gradually increasing. One year back he visited India for medical purpose. Nephrologists there evaluated him and advised renal replacement therapy (RRT). His serum creatinine was 6.5 mg% at that time. He wanted kidney transplantation for which he came to BSMMU. He produced his younger brother as prospective donor. The donor and recipient were thoroughly evaluated. There was zero antigen mismatch. Both donor and recipient were cytomegalovirus (CMV) immunoglobulin G (IgG) positive. The patient did not receive any form of dialysis before. So preemptive renal transplantation was done. Operation was uneventful, warm ischemic time (WIT) was 90 seconds, cold ischemic time (CIT) was 2 hours. There was no immediate post-transplant complication, except a wound dehiscence occurred in the postoperative period and secondary suture was given. Post-transplant weight was 95 kg, blood pressure (BP) was 120/90 mm Hg, and serum creatinine 1.34 mg/dL at discharge.

Afterwards, the patient was on regular follow-up and developed post-transplant diabetes mellitus (PTDM). During the follow-up period, he presented with a history of fever of 1 month duration. The fever was continued type but having an evening rise and associated with chills. Sometimes fever subsided with antipyretic. Had complaints of cough and shortness of breath which were more on exertion, but not associated with any paroxysmal nocturnal dyspnea or orthopnea. He gives history of weight loss of about 6 kg in 2 months. There was no history burning sensation during micturition, headache, abdominal pain, joint pain, skin rash, contact with smear positive pulmonary tuberculosis (TB), travelling to malaria and kala azar endemic zone. On query, his bowel and bladder habit was normal and he was ex-smoker. His father was hypertensive and expired 7 years back, mother is alive and recently diagnosed as DM, other family members are healthy. He was immunized against hepatitis B, *Pneumococcus*, and influenza.

He was taking tablet prednisolone 0.5 mg/kg/day for 3 months, then tapering to a maintenance dose of 5 mg/day, tacrolimus 0.1 mg/kg/day in two divided doses, mycophenolate mofetil 1 g bid, tablet valganciclovir (Valcyte) 450 mg once daily for 3 months, tablet Cotrim 480 mg once daily for 6 months, tablet nifedipine SR 20 mg 1+1+1 to continue, and tablet bisoprolol 5 mg once daily to continue.

On examination, he was obese [body mass index (BMI) 32 kg/m^2], anemia: mild, edema: absent, jaundice: absent, cyanosis: absent, clubbing: absent, skin: some black pigmentation in the limbs, pulse: 100 bpm, carotid bruit: absent, BP: 130/80 mm Hg, temperature: 101°F, respiration: 19 breaths/min, lymph node: not palpable, jugular venous pressure (JVP): not raised, thyroid gland: not enlarged, A functioning arteriovenous (AV) fistula in left forearm, tremor: fine tremor present involving both hands, bedside urine dipstick test: protein—nil, and glucose ++.

Examination of the respiratory system revealed features of left-sided consolidation as evidenced by dull percussion note on the left side from 5th to 9th intercostal space, breath sound—bronchial at the same area. There were crepitations at the same area which were altered with cough, vocal resonance was also increased at the mentioned area.

Gastrointestinal system examination revealed no gum hypertrophy; an oblique scar mark at right iliac fossa, the transplanted kidney is palpable at right iliac fossa, there is no graft tenderness. Liver and spleen were not palpable. There were no ascites, no renal bruit, and fundoscopy revealed grade-2 hypertensive retinopathy.

■ INVESTIGATION (TABLES 1 TO 3)

Urine R/M/E

TABLE 1: Urinalysis.	
Protein	+++
Pus cell	2–5/HPF
RBC	2–5/HPF
Cast	Granular + Cellular +

(RBC: red blood cell)

TABLE 2: Blood count.	
Hb% (g/dL)	9.4
ESR mm in 1st hour	115
TC of WBC	4,500 N-63% L-22%
Platelet	200,000

(ESR: erythrocyte sedimentation rate; RBC: red blood cell; WBC: white blood cell)

TABLE 3: Viral markers.	
HBs Ag	Negative
Anti HCV	Negative
Anti CMV IgM	Negative
Anti CMV IgG	Positive

(CMV: cytomegalovirus; HCV: hepatitis C virus; IgM: immunoglobulin M)

Complete Blood Count

Peripheral blood film:
- RBC—Normocytic normochromic morphology
- WBC—Mature with normal distribution
- Platelet count was normal.

Comment: Normocytic normochromic anemia

Serum creatinine was 1.3 mg/dL at discharge in the post-transplant period.

Chest X-ray posteroanterior (PA) view showed a dense opacity with irregular outer margin in the left zone mid and hilar region with left-sided mild pleural effusion. Cardiac shadow was enlarged in transverse diameter.

Serum electrolyte—Na: 138 mmol/L, K^+:4.1 mmol/L, Cl: 102 mmol/L, TCO_2—26 mmol/L

Blood sugar 2 hours after breakfast was 12 mmol/L, HbA1c: 8.8%, and serum glutamic pyruvic transaminase (SGPT): 14 U/L

Lipid profile—Total cholesterol: 190 mg/dL, high-density lipoprotein (HDL) cholesterol: 28 mg/dL, low-density lipoprotein (LDL) cholesterol: 86 mg/dL, TG: 380 mg/dL, blood urea: 6.2 mmol/L, and uric acid: 365 µmol/L.

Urine C/S: no growth, blood C/S: no growth, sputum C/S: no growth, sputum for acid-fast bacillus (AFB) stain: negative.

Sputum for GeneXpert for MTB—detected, rifampicin resistant (rpoB) gene—not detected

C-reactive protein (CRP): 99 mg/dL (<5 mg/L)

Total iron: 41 µg/dL, total iron-binding capacity (TIBC): 200 µg/dL, transferrin saturation (TSAT): 20%, and serum ferritin: 1,100 ng/mL
Ultrasonography (USG) of transplant kidney
- Transplant kidney is normal in size.
- Bipolar length is 10.0 cm.
- Cortex and medulla are well-defined; pelvicalyceal system is not dilated.

▋ DISCUSSION

Our patient undergone preemptive renal transplantation. Studies show that patient who is transplanted preemptively carries an advantage compared with a patient who has needed long-time dialysis before transplantation and there is also a significant improvement in graft survival. And the longer the period of dialysis before transplantation, the worse the outcome.

He was put on triple immunosuppression viz. prednisolone, mycophenolate mofetil, and tacrolimus. Tacrolimus is more potent as immunosuppressive drug compared to cyclosporine, although the mechanism of action is same. But tacrolimus is more diabetogenic then cyclosporine. Our patient developed PTDM, which might have association with tacrolimus.

The current patient presented with pulmonary TB during follow-up period and he was put on anti-TB chemotherapy which included rifampicin. There is a drug–drug interaction between tacrolimus and rifampicin, threatening transplanted organ with rejection or TB with treatment failure. The interaction leads to decrease tacrolimus levels and may increase the risk of rejection which we had to manage by increasing dose of tacrolimus to reach therapeutic levels.

FREQUENTLY ASKED QUESTIONS

Q1. What is preemptive transplantation?

Ans. Chronic kidney disease patient when undergo transplantation before starting dialysis treatment—it is called preemptive transplantation.

Q2. What are the benefits of preemptive transplantation?

Ans.
- The risk of rejection is less
- Could avoid dialysis with avoiding dialysis related complications
- Better patient survival
- Better graft survival

Q3. What are the risk factors for PTDM?

Ans.

- Family history of DM
- Age >40 years
- Human leukocyte antigen (HLA) A30 B27 B42
- HLA mismatch
- Pre-transplant impaired glucose tolerance (IGT)
- CMV infection
- Calcineurin inhibitor (CNI)
- Steroid
- Mammalian target of rapamycin (mTOR) inhibitor

Acute Kidney Injury

▮ INTRODUCTION

Mr AL, a 26-year-old businessman, was referred to the Department of Nephrology, Bangabandhu Sheikh Mujib Medical University (BSMMU), Dhaka, for management of acute renal failure. He complained of severe body ache following recent incidence of unaccustomed physical exercise, thereafter being treated by the local physician with nonsteroidal anti-inflammatory drugs (NSAIDs). Although his pain was alleviated but 2 days later, he noticed reduced volume of urine and became confused and then admitted to local hospital. There was no history of fever, joint pain, or rash. He has given history of going to gymnasium 3 days ago where he undergone heavy physical exercise. He was not used to regular exercise before this episode. He did three rounds of squats 20 each, then he was introduced to weight training exercises of lower body such as leg press, leg curl, leg extension, and adduction-abduction. He did them for about 40 minutes. Then, he did cardio for 15 minutes in the form of static cycling. Then, before cooling down, he did 20 crunches (abdominals). He had a lot of muscle pain postexercise, which he ignored for some time. He was not on any medications or any performance-enhancing substances. He was not doing any exercise for previous 2 years. There was no history of similar attack in the past. His urine output dropped and blood investigations showed higher creatinine; hence, he was shifted to tertiary care hospital. His vital was normal. Examination showed tenderness and swelling in both arm and thigh muscle groups. Movements were painful. There was no ecchymosis and no sensory or motor deficit of the limbs. Distal arterial pulsation were normal. His laboratory parameters were: Hemoglobin (Hb) 13.5 g/dL, total leukocyte count 8,100 m^3, platelets 2.15 K, urine analysis showed albumin: 3+, red blood cell: 0–2/high power field (HPF), white blood cell (WBC): 1–2/HPF, and granular casts: 6–8/HPF. Creatinine phosphokinase: 29,000, lactate dehydrogenase (LDH): 10,100, uric acid: 10.8, serum sodium:

131 mEq/L, potassium: 5.9 mEq/L, blood urea nitrogen: 35 mg/dL, and serum creatinine: 12.9 mg/dL. On admission, there was metabolic acidosis with pH: 7.27 and pCO_2: 28. Myoglobin levels were not assessed. Ultrasound abdomen showed bilateral increased renal cortical echogenicity with loss of corticomedullary differentiation. Rest of the study within normal limits. Magnetic resonance imaging of the leg or paraumbilical muscles was not undertaken due to cost constraints. Echocardiogram showed normal functioning heart. A diagnosis of acute kidney injury (AKI) secondary to rhabdomyolysis was made. Patient was treated with several session of hemodialysis through left femoral venous catheter and his urine output returned to normal after 9 days. He was discharged with serum creatinine 1.1 mg/dL.

DISCUSSION

Rhabdomyolysis is a common clinical condition resulting from a wide variety of physical and nonphysical causes. Most common causes are trauma that occurs in accidents or assault. Others result from strenuous exercise, status epilepticus, delirium tremens, high voltage electrical injury, and hyperthermia. Various myopathies, myositis, electrolyte imbalances, and systemic infections such as toxic shock syndrome, falciparum malaria, leptospirosis, and legionellosis are among the nonphysical causes which contribute to rhabdomyolysis. Rhabdomyolysis can results from envenomation also, there were some reports that bee sting could be one of the important causes of renal failure due to rhabdomyolysis. Strenuous muscular exercise causes myolysis especially in untrained individuals and in individuals exercising in hot and humid conditions. It is also very well known that heat stress as in malignant hyperthermia causes myolysis.

In this case, our young patient presented with classic sings of rhabdomyolysis. He is healthy and this is the first time of hospitalization for him. He is not on any performance-enhancing drugs. He did strenuous exercise on the very first day of gym in his youthful enthusiasm. He sought medical treatment after 24 hours. He received nonsteroidal anti-inflammatory medication for his severe musculoskeletal pain. He did not hydrate himself well after exercise. Excessive eccentric exercise of leg, arm, and abdominal muscles posed him to land into rhabdomyolysis. All these factors that is, eccentric muscle damage, late treatment, dehydration, and nephrotoxic insult by NSAIDs, must have caused the renal insufficiency with which he presented. Eccentric muscle damage response can be more stressed in individuals that are susceptible toward exertional rhabdo-myolysis (high responders). Squats, push-ups, static cycling with resistance done on machine are the examples of eccentric exercise.

Myoglobinuria does not occur without rhabdomyolysis. Myoglobulin is rapidly and unpredictably cleared by hepatic metabolism. Therefore, test for myoglobulin in plasma or urine is not a sensitive diagnostic tool. It is also readily filtered by glomeruli. Water is progressively reabsorbed and the concentration of myoglobin rises proportionately, until it precipitates and causes obstructive cast formation and thus AKI. Release of myoglobulin is often associated with an increase in levels of creatine kinase (CK), aldolase, LDH, serum glutamic-pyruvic transaminase, and other enzymes. Because overall degradation and removal of CK is slow, its concentration remains elevated much longer and in a more consistent manner than that of myoglobin. Consequently, CK is more reliable than myoglobin is assessing the presence and intensity of damage to the muscle. There was no defined threshold value of serum CK above which the risk of AKI is markedly increased. The risk of AKI in rhabdomyolysis is usually low when CK levels at admission are <15000–20,000 U/L. Although AKI may be associated with CK values as low as 5,000 U/L, this usually occurs when coexisting conditions such as sepsis, dehydration, and acidosis are present. Our patient had CK of 29,000 on admission. The true incidence of AKI in rhabdomyolysis is difficult to establish owing to varying definitions and clinical scenarios. The reported incidence ranges from 13% to approximately 50%. Acute kidney injury associated with rhabdomyolysis often leads to a more rapid increase in plasma creatinine than do other forms of AKI as seen in our patient. Similarly, a low ratio of blood urea nitrogen to creatinine is often seen in patients with rhabdomyolysis. Rhabdomyolysis-induced AKI frequently causes oliguria and occasionally causes anuria. The outcome of rhabdomyolysis is usually good provided that there is no renal failure. Nevertheless, mortality data vary widely according to the study population, setting, the number and severity of coexisting conditions. Among patients in intensive care unit (ICU), the mortality has been reported to be 59% when AKI is present and 22% when it is not present.

Long-term survival among patients with rhabdomyolysis and AKI is reported to be close to 80% and the majority of patients recover renal function.

FREQUENTLY ASKED QUESTIONS

Q1. What is non-traumatic rhabdomyolysis?

Ans. It can occur in extreme exertion or normal physical exertion in addition to risk factors that impair muscle oxygenation. Conditions which are associated with non-traumatic rhabdomyolysis are seizures, heat illness, drugs (e.g., statins), infection, electrolyte imbalance, etc.

Q2. What are the symptoms triad of rhabdomyolysis?

Ans.

- Muscle pain
- Muscle weakness
- Dark red/brown urine or decreased urination

Q3. What are the laboratory parameters for diagnosis of rhabdomyolysis?

Ans.

- Serum CK (~1,000 U/L) or five times upper limit of normal (ULN)
- Serum glutamic oxaloacetic transaminase (SGOT)
- Serum glutamic pyruvic transaminase (SGPT)
- LDH
- Blood and urine myoglobin test

Q4. What are the Acute Kidney Injury Network (AKIN) criteria of AKI?

Ans. Acute Kidney Injury Network (AKIN) defines AKI as:

- *Stage 1*: An absolute increase in serum creatinine of 0.3 mg/dL (26 μmol/L) or greater or a 50–100% increase from baseline. Urine output <0.5 mL/kg/h × 6 hours.
- *Stage 2*: Serum creatinine >2 mg/dL or serum creatinine ≤3 mg/dL × baseline. Urine output <0.5 mL/kg/h × 12 hours.
- *Stage 3*: Serum creatinine >3 mg/dL × baseline or serum creatinine >4 mg/dL with an acute rise ≥0.5 mg/dL or on renal replacement therapy (RRT).

Q5. Urinary finding in rhabdomyolysis?

Ans. Urine test strip is positive for blood but contains no red blood cell (RBC) on microscopic examination.

Gitelman Syndrome

▌ INTRODUCTION

A 18-year-old male patient with persistent hypokalemia was referred by internist to the nephrologist. This condition has first been found at the age of 17 years during hospitalization for tingling sensation of upper and lower limb for one and half months, muscle spasm of both upper and lower limb with perioral paresthesia for 2–3 days.

He was diagnosed as a case of diabetes mellitus (DM), hypertension (HTN), and ankylosing spondylitis and was getting treatment for those conditions.

He suffered from polyuria and nocturia with no other urinary tract symptoms. None of his family members suffered from such type of illness.

On physical examination, he had blood pressure of 130/90 mm Hg and regular pulse rate of 88 bpm, normal hydration, and coloration of skin and mucosa. Cardiopulmonary examination was normal with no signs of dependent edema. The remaining physical examination was normal.

On arterial blood gas analysis, he had metabolic alkalosis (pH 7.54; pCO_2 42.4 mm Hg; HCO_3 34.1 mmol/L). Biochemical analysis revealed hypokalemia (2.5 mmol/L), hypomagnesemia (1.2 mmol/L), and hypochloremia (95 mmol/L); serum calcium 7.3 mg/dL, 24 hours urinary analysis revealed decreased excretion of calcium (0.5 mmol/24 hours), serum creatinine 90 μmol/L, urea 6.3 mmol/L, further investigation revealed plasma-active rennin 9 pg/mL (4.4–46.1), serum aldosterone 62 pg/mL (30–400 pg/mL), hypocalciuria: 0.5 mmol/day (2.5–7.5), and urinary excretion of sodium 213 mmol/L (40–220), and chloride 247 mmol/L (110–250). Estimated glomerular filtrate rate [modification of diet in renal disease (MDRD)] was 103.23 mL/min/1.73 m². Electrocardiogram showed normal sinus rhythm with a heart rate of 74 bpm. Renal ultrasound and renal and adrenal computed tomography (CT) revealed normal findings.

A limitation to this case report was that the diagnosis could not be ascertained with sequencing of the implicated gene due to unavailability of genetic sequencing at the facility, i.e., Bangabandhu Sheikh Mujib Medical University.

■ DISCUSSION

In 1966, Gitelman et al. described a familial disorder in three adult female patients with occasional episodes of muscle weakness and tetany. Neither growth retardation nor polyuria was detected. Hypokalemia, hypomagnesemia, and hypocalciuria were present. This familial disorder was named as Gitelman syndrome (GS) and diagnosis was based on these clinical and biochemical findings.

The prevalence of GS is estimated at approximately 1 in 40,000 and accordingly the prevalence of people heterozygous for the condition is approximately 1% in Caucasian population. However, there is paucity of data about the clinical variability and carrier rate in other populations. GS usually presents after the age of 6 years and mostly the diagnosis is made only in adulthood. In our patient, the symptoms started at the age of 27 years in the form of recurrent episodes of muscle weakness.

As described before, we postulate that GS can present in early childhood with milder symptoms and become fully symptomatic in adolescence. In our patient, disease manifested at the age of 27 years.

Gitelman syndrome is an autosomal recessive trait. It is caused by missense mutation in the *SLC12A3* gene (located on chromosome 16q) that encodes the thiazide-sensitive sodium chloride cotransporter. In SLC12A3, 172 distinct mutations have been described, leading to extreme phenotype variability. Female patients with the same mutations are relatively asymptomatic compared with their male counterparts. The nature and position of the SLC12A3 mutation, combined with male gender, seem to be a determinant factor in the severity of GS. Defects in the thiazide-sensitive sodium chloride cotransporter in the distal convoluted tubule (DCT) impair sodium and chloride reabsorption in that tubule, causing natriuresis and leading to mild volume contraction. This volume contraction and increased sodium delivery to the macula densa activates the renin–angiotensin–aldosterone axis. Aldosterone increases sodium reabsorption in the cortical collecting duct and leads to increased secretion of potassium and hydrogen ions. This caused hypokalemia and alkalosis. Nijenhuis et al. demonstrated hypocalciuria and hypomagnesemia in mouse models for GS and chronic thiazide diuretic use. Hypocalciuria was secondary to the downregulation of magnesium channels (TRPM6) in the DCT.

Most patients present with muscle cramps, weakness, paresthesias, and episodes of tetany or paralysis. Almost 6% of patients experience hypokalemic paralysis, similar to our patient; other symptoms include nocturia, polydipsia, diarrhea, dizziness, and salt craving. These symptoms are attributed to the electrolyte and acid–base abnormalities. The most of patients also develop hypotension. GS can sometimes cause short stature and growth failures. In case of our patient, there is no history of growth retardation or no history of hypotension. This may be due to delayed onset of disease.

Hypokalemia and hypomagnesemia lead to a prolonged QT interval in >50% of patients with GS. However, cardiac arrhythmias have been described in fewer patients. Sudden cardiac death has been reported in few cases.

A diagnosis of GS is based on clinical findings and biochemical abnormalities. Typical laboratory findings include hypokalemia, metabolic alkalosis, hypomagnesemia, and hypocalciuria. Alongside other renal salt-wasting syndromes (such as Bartter syndrome), GS is considered to be a rare cause of hypokalemic metabolic alkalosis. However, the distinguishing features of GS are hypomagnesemia and hypocalciuria.

Treatment is directed at correcting potassium and magnesium depletion. It requires lifelong liberal salt intake. Potassium supplementation is with potassium chloride and potassium-sparing diuretics, including amiloride and spironolactone. However, in hypotensive patients, these drugs should be used with caution. Hypomagnesemia is corrected with magnesium chloride (magnesium sulfate or oxide are avoided to prevent diarrhea).

FREQUENTLY ASKED QUESTIONS

Q1. How can you differentiate between Bartter and Gitelman?

Ans. Children with Bartter syndrome commonly demonstrate hypercalciuria with normal serum magnesium, whereas Gitelman syndrome typically show hypocalciuria and hypomagnesemia.

Q2. Why is potassium and magnesium low in Gitelman syndrome?

Ans. Hypokalemia is due to activation of renin–angiotensin system due to loss of NaCl cotransporter (NCCT) function.

Hypomagnesemia is due to renal magnesium wasting caused by down-regulation of epithelial Mg channel TRPM6 in DCT.

Q3. How do you get Gitelman syndrome?

Ans. It is an autosomal recessive disorder. Gitelman syndrome is usually caused by mutation in *SLC12A3* gene. It may also result from mutation in *CLCNKB* gene. The proteins produced from these genes are involved in kidneys reabsorption of salt (NaCl).

Renal Amyloidosis

▮ INTRODUCTION

Mrs AK 42-year-old female with history of sudden light-headedness, headache, slurring of speech along with left-sided weakness 6 months ago and admitted in a specialized hospital and diagnosed as hypertension, ischemic stroke with left-sided hemiparesis, and was treated accordingly and discharged in a stable state. Re-admitted with altered consciousness and labeled as urosepsis and treated conservatively with parenteral antibiotic. While on treatment, patient developed generalized swelling without any apparent change in urine color or volume and was found to have nephrotic range proteinuria. She was referred to nephrologist for further evaluation and management. She is hypertensive for last 4 years. She has no history of sore throat, skin rash, joint pain or oral ulcer, chest pain, breathlessness, jaundice, cold intolerance, weight loss, and bowel abnormality. Gives no history of taking any herbal medicine or nephrotoxic drug. She had pitting bipedal edema extending up to the knee and had pallor, but no jaundice, clubbing, or any organomegaly. Vitals are within normal limit.

Her urine for routine and microscopic examination showed albumin +++, white blood cell (WBC) 10–12/high power field (HPF), red blood cell 2–3/ HPF with a significant growth of *Enterobacter* in culture. 24-hour urinary protein was 8.6 g. Complete blood count revealed hemoglobin 9.2 g/dL, erythrocyte sedimentation rate 80 mm in 1st hour, WBC 16,500/cmm and out of which polymorphs 80%, lymphocyte 17%, eosinophils 0, monocytes 3%, and basophils 1% with normal platelet count. Other blood reports were— serum creatinine 1.8 mg/dL (initially), then 1.2 mg/dL [after treatment of urinary tract infection (UTI)], total protein 55 g/L, serum albumin 23 g/L, calcium 9 mg/dL, phosphate 3 mg/dL, parathyroid hormone 39 pg/mL, uric acid 8.3 mg/dL, and cholesterol 325 mg/dL. She has normal blood sugar, liver function, and thyroid function. Serum complements C3 and C4 were normal, antinuclear antibody (ANA), antids-DNA, and antineutrophil cytoplasmic antibodies (ANCAs) were negative. Viral screen including antihuman immunodeficiency virus (HIV) 1 and 2, hepatitis B surface antigen, and anti-hepatitis C virus antibody were negative. Radiological investigations such as plain X-ray of kidney, ureter, and bladder (KUB), chest X-ray posteroanterior (P/A) view, and X-ray skull B/V were normal. Ultrasonography of whole abdomen showed slightly bigger kidneys (right kidney—12.5 × 5.3 cm, left kidney 13 × 5.5 cm) with increased cortical echogenicity. She has normal electrocardiography and echocardiography. Myeloma screen (**Tables 1 and 2**) including serum protein electrophoresis and immunofixation study showed no "M" spike with normal kappa and lambda (κ/λ) ratio of 0.73 on serum free light chain assay and urinary Bence Jones protein was negative. Her renal biopsy demonstrated congophilic amyloid deposition in glomeruli, interstitium and blood vessel wall which displayed apple-green birefringence with polarizer, and these deposition had 3+ lamda positivity. These results led to the diagnosis of amyloidosis, AL type. She was referred to hematology and her bone marrow examination was performed which showed significant increased plasma cells (about 10%). Now patient is getting chemotherapy (bortezomib 0.7 mg/m^2 body surface area and dexamethasone 40 mg/day) under the supervision of hematologist.

TABLE 1: Serum free light chains.

Kappa and lambda light chains, free, serum @ (nephelometry)	Results	Units	Bio, ref, interval
Kappa, free light chain	84.70	mg/L	3.30–19.40
Lambda, free light chain	116.00	mg/L	5.71–26.30
Kappa and lambda, ratio	0.730		0.26–1.65

TABLE 2: Serum protein electrophoresis.

Protein electrophoresis, serum @ (capillary electrophoresis)	Results	Units	
Total protein	5.90	g/dL	6.40–8.30
Albumin	2.60	g/dL	3.60–5.50
Alpha 1 globulin	0.35	g/dL	0.20–0.40
Alpha 2 globulin	0.92	g/dL	0.50–1.00
Beta 1 globulin	0.25	g/dL	0.50–1.10
Beta 2 globulin	0.41	g/dL	0.30–0.60
Gamma globulin	1.37	g/dL	0.70–1.60
A:G Ratio	0.79		0.90–2.00
M. Spike	Not seen	g/dL	

▇ BONE MARROW EXAMINATION REPORT

Plasma cells: Bone marrow is occupied by some plasma cells with various stages of development (about 10%).

Renal Biopsy

Microscopic Description

Multiple step serial sections from renal core stained with hematoxylin and eosin (H&E), periodic acid–Schiff (PAS), Masson's trichrome (MT), and periodic Schiff-methenamine (PASM) show 17 glomeruli, four of them are obsolescent.

Glomeruli

All of them show pale eosinophilic acellular, weak PAS-positive material in the mesangial and basement membrane, focally forming nodules. It is silver-positive, congophilic, and displays apple-green birefringence with polarizer (Congo-red stain). There is no necrotizing lesion or crescent formation.

Tubules/Interstitium

Similar acellular amyloid material is seen focally along the tubular basement membranes and in the interstitial space. There are foci of moderate degree of atrophic tubules. There is no focus of interstitial inflammation or eosinophils or granuloma.

Vessels

There is amyloid deposit in the wall of interlobular arteries and arterioles. Congo-red stain is positive for amyloid.

Immunofluorescence

Four viable glomeruli are seen. Glomerular tufts are negative for granular deposits with panel of antisera [immunoglobulin G (IgG), IgA, IgM, C3, C1q]. κ/λ light chain stains show restriction of one of them, in the form of lambda (3+) positivity in the amyloid deposits seen in glomeruli and vessels. Kappa light chain is negative in these areas.

Impression

Kidney biopsy:
- Amyloidosis, AL type (lambda light-chain restriction)
- *Additional features*: Focal global glomerulosclerosis (25%), moderate tubular atrophy, and interstitial fibrosis (30–40%)

▇ DISCUSSION

Amyloidosis may be systemic or localized. The most common presentation of primary amyloidosis is nephrotic syndrome (which was present in our case), chronic heart failure, hepatosplenomegaly, carpal tunnel syndrome, etc. Coexisting symptoms of multiple myeloma can sometimes help in diagnosis. Kidney and heart involvements are the major causes of death. Almost every patient with AL amyloidosis has clonal B-cell dysplasia, but none of widely available laboratory tests using blood or urine samples, as well as none of imaging studies specific enough to determine the certain diagnosis of amyloidosis independently of other examinations results.

According to diagnostic criteria of the Mayo Clinic, to recognize systemic light-chain amyloidosis we need to reveal coexistence of the following findings:
- Clinical symptoms resulting from amyloid infiltration of particular organs
- Positive result of amyloid Congo red staining in biopsy material containing amyloid deposits
- Evidence indicating that amyloid deposits contain immunoglobulin light chains proteins
- Confirmed presence of monoclonal plasma cell proliferative disorder

It was estimated that about 2–3% of patient suffering from AL amyloidosis do not meet above criteria of diagnosis. A patient with clinically suspected AL amyloidosis, serum and urine immunofixation along with Ig-free light chain (FLC) assay should be used as screening tools. Sensitivity of serum electrophoresis is 71%, urine electrophoresis is 84%, and circulating FLCs measurements reach 98%, nevertheless their specificity is low as they give false positive results in the case of other types of plasma cell dyscrasias. In healthy individuals, prevalence of κ light chains in bone marrow is observed, while in patients with AL amyloidosis κ/λ FLC ratio 1:30 is a characteristic feature. It is assumed that the normal value of κ/λ ratio makes the diagnosis of AL amyloidosis unlikely. In our patient, despite the finally achieved definitive confirmation of AL amyloidosis, κ/λ ratio measured during hospitalization was 0.73 with the reference of the normal range from 0.26 to 1.65. Ultrasonography in renal amyloidosis typically shows enlarged kidneys, which was present in our case. The next diagnostic step is tissue biopsy for amyloid protein detection. Tissue samples usually undergo Congo red staining. It enables obtaining pathognomonic green birefringence of stained tissues examined under polarized light in the case of amyloid deposit in the tissue specimen. The choice of biopsy site seems to be another essential issue. Theoretically, knowing which of the patient's organ is affected, we are able to use biopsy to get a tissue sample directly from the diseased organ expecting high reliability of such targeted biopsy procedure. Indeed, it has been estimated that amyloid accumulation can be visualized in >90% of liver or kidney biopsies taken from patients with AL amyloidosis. However, attention should be paid to the fact that biopsy of organ poses in particular a risk of internal bleeding. So it seems to be reasonable to treat parenchymatous organ biopsy rather as the procedure of last choice, which can be used when other, less invasive methods give equivocal results. A simple and safe method with a relatively high sensitivity (60–80%) is the biopsy of subcutaneous fatty tissue. Biopsies of rectal mucosa and bone marrow are also often used, the sensitivity of these is 50–70% and 50–55%, respectively.

FREQUENTLY ASKED QUESTIONS

Q1. What are the different types of amyloidosis?

Ans.

- *AL amyloidosis (immunoglobulin light chain amyloidosis)*: It is also called primary amyloidosis.
- AA amyloidosis also known as secondary amyloidosis, this condition is the result of another chronic infections or inflammatory disease such as Crohn's disease and rheumatoid arthritis.
- *Dialysis-related amyloidosis*: People who have been on dialysis for 5 years or more may develop this. There is deposition of beta 2 microglobulin in bones, joints, tendons, etc.
- *Familial or hereditary amyloidosis*: Many genetic defects are linked.

Q2. How renal amyloidosis is diagnosed?

Ans. Renal biopsy and histologic demonstration of amyloid deposits by staining with Congo red dye. Congo red stained amyloid has an orange red appearance under light microscopy and produces apple green birefringence under polarized light.

Q3. How is dialysis related Amyloidosis is treated?

Ans.

- Use of newer hemodialysis filter to reduce amyloid protein levels in blood
- Surgery for conditions such as carpal tunnel syndrome
- Kidney transplantation

Q4. What is the newer treatment of renal amyloidosis?

Ans. Isatuximab, a monoclonal antibody approved for treatment of multiple myeloma, can effectively treat relapsed and refractory AL amyloidosis.

Note: The examinee may be asked to demonstrate ballottement of kidney.

Down's Syndrome with Chronic Kidney Disease

◼ INTRODUCTION

The patient, a 25-year-old female, was diagnosed as a case of Down's syndrome (DS) based on clinical features by a pediatrician in her early childhood. Despite being a DS patient, she had been in surprisingly good physical state other than bowel bladder incontinence. However, she was almost completely dependent on others for most of her daily household activities, as reflected in her Waisman Activities of Daily Living (W-ADL) score of 2 out of 34.

One month ago, her father noticed that she was not eating well, felling weak, and was less responsive than usual. The symptoms continued for 4 more days; by that time, she became progressively weaker, developed vomiting, and suddenly collapsed at one point. She was taken to the hospital, labeled as septicemia, and later shifted to an intensive care unit (ICU) due to deterioration of her condition. During ICU stay, she developed decreased urinary output, dependent edema, and respiratory distress and her serum creatinine was found to be raised. At that point, she was transferred to the department of nephrology.

During our evaluation at nephrology department, it was found that she is drowsy and afebrile. She had persistently raised blood pressure of around 140/90 mm Hg, facial puffiness, dependent edema, and a urinary output of about 750–1,000 mL/day. She displayed several phenotypical features of DS, such as epicanthic eye-fold, low-set ears, downturned corners of mouth, flat face, protruding tongue, and general hypotonia. Although these criteria have shown to lead to successful clinical diagnosis of DS in newborns, they had to be relied upon in this instance since no such clinical criteria were available for the diagnosis of DS in adults. Her father denied any history of skin rash, oral ulcer, photosensitivity, joint pain, jaundice, or history of blood transfusion. She had an episode of possible gastroenteritis 1 month prior to this illness, but it resolved spontaneously without any apparent residual affect.

The laboratory examination reports are: Her urine routine examination showed +3 proteinuria, red blood cell (RBC) 30–40/high power field (HPF). Urine and blood cultures revealed no growth. Serum creatinine was 15 mg/dL at presentation. Abdominal ultrasonogram revealed bilateral small sized kidneys (right 6.78 × 3.58 cm, left 8.02 × 3.23 cm), cortical echogenicity was increased, but corticomedullary differentiation (CMD) was well-maintained. Echocardiography revealed no abnormalities.

She had received multiple intravenous antibiotics during her ICU stay. She was labeled as a case of chronic kidney disease (CKD) stage 5 and advised immediate renal replacement therapy (RRT). Thrice weekly hemodialysis (HD) was started through a temporary central venous (femoral) catheter. After a week of dialysis, her serum creatinine came down to and became somewhat stable at around 5 mg/dL. Other general treatment measures for CKD were taken.

Several investigations, such as karyotyping, micturating cystourethrogram (MCUG), dimercaptosuccinic acid (DMSA) scan, abdominal CT scan, and renal biopsy were discussed to determine the underlying etiology of her renal condition. But after understanding the irreversible nature of her condition and knowing that these procedures would have limited effect on her future management, these investigations were not done. The prospect of future renal transplantation was also denied due to financial constraints. With a wife diagnosed as a case of major depressive disorder and a high caregiver burden (42 out of 88 on Zarit Burden Interview, Bangla), his (father of the patient) decision was understandable and respected by our colleagues.

■ DISCUSSION

Our patient presented with renal impairment along with uremic features. Though her presentation was acute, a low serum calcium and small sized kidneys point toward CKD. It is unlikely that the episode of gastroenteritis had acted as an acute insult on a preexisting CKD, since she was asymptomatic in the interim period. Previous studies support this with the evidence that the risk of dehydration is not increased in DS patients with diarrhea compared to non-DS diarrhea patients.

Since extensive imaging studies or renal biopsy could not be performed, we can only speculate about the conditions leading to CKD in this case. Ultrasonography revealed that despite both kidneys being small, the CMD was well-maintained. This could be due to congenital renal hypoplasia. Along with the hematuria and proteinuria, secondary focal segmental glomerulosclerosis (FSGS) due to hyperfiltration injury could have led to end-stage renal disease (ESRD). Since vesicoureteral reflux (VUR) is one of the urinary tract anomalies found in DS, which can also explain the urinary incontinence in our patient, VUR-induced FSGS, chronic pyelonephritis, or chronic tubulointerstitial disease could be other possible explanation of ESRD in this case. Since obtaining renal biopsy is difficult in DS patients, studies regarding primary glomerulonephritis (GN) in DS are rare. A few cases have been reported, with immunoglobulin A (IgA) nephropathy and FSGS proving to be the most common forms of GN. However, a significant predilection toward any primary GN was not noted.

The presence of renal involvement was not considered to be a common phenomenon in DS previously. Consequently, routine screening for renal function or urological anomalies have not been recommended by authorities such as the 2011 American Academy of Pediatrics guidelines. In recent years, an increasing number of studies are showing quite high prevalence of renal and urinary tract abnormalities (RUTAs) in patients with DS ranging from 3.2 to 21.2%, especially after the second and third decades. Among the DS patients with RUTAs, ESRD is not an uncommon outcome.

This study has several limitations. The diagnosis of DS was made based on clinical signs; karyotyping could not be performed. Imaging studies that could have helped shed more light on establishing the underlying etiology of the ESRD could not be done. No Bangla version of the W-ADL questionnaire was available. It had to be executed on a version translated by the author, so testing for external, internal, or construct validities was not possible. The Zarit Burden interview on the other hand has been previously translated in Bangla and tested for validity.

This case shows us that kidney diseases in DS patients often go unnoticed in our community. It is possible to perform and maintain regular HD in patient with DS. With increasing survival of people with DS, there is increased prevalence of RUTAs that needs screening and regular follow-up of renal function.

FREQUENTLY ASKED QUESTIONS

Q1. **What are the kidney problems that can occur in Down's syndrome (DS) patient?**

Ans. Kidney disease is not a frequent problem in DS patient. But a variety problems such as voiding disturbances, mild hydronephrosis, hyperuricosuria, hyperuricemia without gout, mild proteinuria, microscopic hematuria, and CKD can occur in DS patients.

Q2. **Which type of dialysis treatment is suitable for patients of Down's syndrome (DS) with ESKD?**

Ans. Peritoneal dialysis is not suitable for DS with ESKD because of lack of cooperation and hence increased risk of peritonitis.

Continuous Ambulatory Peritoneal Dialysis Peritonitis

▍INTRODUCTION

Mrs MA, a 57-year-old housewife, was diagnosed as a case of hypertension, chronic stable angina, and renal impairment 8 years ago. Her serum creatinine was found to be 1.8 mg/dL. Although she had good compliance to medications and hypertension was well-controlled, renal function progressively deteriorated and serum creatinine rose to 8.1 mg/dL over the next 9 months. She was labeled as a case of chronic kidney disease (CKD) and advised for renal replacement therapy (RRT) in the form of hemodialysis (HD). HD was successfully started via arteriovenous fistula (AVF) and continued for 10 months. Since she lived over 100 km away from the closest HD facility, she switched to continuous ambulatory peritoneal dialysis (CAPD) at that point.

She initially received three daily exchanges of 2 L. Two years ago, she started experiencing volume overload and was switched to four daily exchanges, which lead to resolution of her symptoms. She alternated between 1.5 and 2.5% dextrose solutions. She did not experience any episodes of persistent abdominal pain along with cloudy effluent and/or peritoneal dialysis (PD) catheter site redness or tenderness.

She presented with a history of abdominal pain and cloudy PD effluent for 10 days. The pain was gradual in onset, diffuse, not associated with any radiation, had no relationship with food intake, or any aggravating or relieving factors. It was associated with anorexia, nausea, and occasional vomiting. The PD effluent was cloudy, but not hemorrhagic. It was initially associated with redness and tenderness of the skin overlying the PD catheter tunnel. There was no associated drain pain. CAPD fluid examination revealed:

- *Cytology*: White blood cell (WBC)—500/mm^3 (90% neutrophils) and red blood cell (RBC)—100/mm^3

- *Sugar*: 30.2 mmol/L and protein—218 mg/dL
- *Acid-fast bacillus (AFB)*: Not found
- *GeneXpert*: Not detected
- *Culture sensitivity*: *Mycobacterium tuberculosis (MTB)* No growth

She was put on empirical intraperitoneal vancomycin and ceftazidime for 21 days, which did not lead to any improvement in symptoms or effluent color. She was labeled as a case of refractory peritonitis and PD catheter was removed. Jugular catheterization was done and HD was initiated. AVF construction was done.

She was kept nothing by mouth and given periodic nasogastric suction along with parenteral nutrition. Her abdominal pain lessened in intensity, but anorexia, nausea, occasional vomiting, and severe constipation persisted. Bowel moved only twice with small volume stool, despite multiple forms of laxatives and enemas.

On examination, abdomen was diffusely tender, with a soft, firm mass present beneath the catheter removal site. Bowel sound was present. Abdominal ultrasonogram revealed bilaterally symmetrically contracted kidneys measuring 7.1 and 6.1 cm and ascites. Computed tomography (CT) scan of abdomen was done, which revealed ascites, bowel wall thickening, and few peritoneal calcifications.

Surgical and gastroenterological consultation was taken and they advised to continue conservative management for the gastrointestinal complains, with a plan of surgical intervention in mind if she showed no improvement. She eventually discharged herself from the hospital against our best medical advice.

DISCUSSION

Peritonitis is a common and severe complication in PD. When a patient on PD presents with clinical features compatible with PD-associated peritonitis, empirical antibiotic therapy with coverage of both gram-positive and gram-negative organisms, should be started; once the appropriate microbiological specimens are collected.

Intraperitoneal route is the preferred route of antibiotic administration. Antifungal prophylaxis with oral nystatin should be added. Once the PD effluent Gram-stain or culture and sensitivity results are available—the antibiotic may be adjusted. The duration of antibiotics is usually 2–3 weeks.

Catheter removal and temporary HD support is recommended for refractory, relapsing, or fungal peritonitis. In some patients, new PD catheter could be inserted after complete resolution of peritonitis. After catheter removal for fungal or refractory peritonitis, effective antibiotics should be continued for another 2 weeks.

Peritoneal dialysis catheter should also be removed for refractory exit site or tunnel infection. Prompt treatment of exit site and catheter infection are key measures to prevent PD-associated peritonitis.

FREQUENTLY ASKED QUESTIONS

Q1. How do you diagnose PD peritonitis?

Ans. Any two of the following:

- Clinical features of peritonitis, i.e., abdominal pain or cloudy dialysis effluent
- Dialysis effluent WBC count >100/μL with >50% neutrophils
- Positive dialysis effluent culture
- Gram-staining of PD effluent also helps diagnosis

Q2. What is refractory peritonitis?

Ans. Failure of clearance of peritoneal fluid despite 5 days of appropriate antibiotic therapy.

Q3. What are the measures to prevent PD peritonitis?

Ans.

- Prophylactic antibiotics before PD catheter insertion, colonoscopy, or invasive gynecologic procedures
- Daily topical application of antibiotic cream/ointment to the catheter exit site
- Prompt treatment of exit site/catheter infection

Note: The examinee may be asked to show steps of handwashing before performing PD exchanges.

Wilson's Disease with Focal Segmental Glomerulosclerosis

■ INTRODUCTION

Mr H, an 18-year-old nondiabetic, normotensive student, presented to us with a history of generalized swelling for 1 year. A diagnosis of nephrotic syndrome was made based on urinary total protein (UTP) of 4.7 g/day with bland urine sediment. He did not have any other symptoms.

He was prescribed high-dose prednisolone (2 mg/kg every alternate day). It was continued for 6 months. He achieved partial remission, UTP coming down to 1.7 g/day. After discontinuation of steroid, his UTP rose to 10.1 g/day over a course of 6 months and serum creatinine started to rise. Highest serum creatinine was 2.4 mg/dL. Suspecting steroid dependence, we decided to perform renal biopsy. Unfortunately, biopsy yielded only four glomeruli (inadequate specimen), and revealed mild mesangial proliferation and is focally prominent glomerular basement membrane (GBM).

He was put on oral mycophenolate mofetil (MMF) 3 g/day. After continuing this treatment for two and a half months, UTP and serum creatinine came down to 2.1 g/day and 1.4 mg/dL.

Interestingly, over the course of this 1 year, although his UTP fluctuated between 1.7 and 10.1 g/day, his serum albumin remained persistently low, ranging from 9 to 15 g/L. He did not give any history of diarrhea, steatorrhea, or jaundice. Consultations with gastroenterologist, nephrologist, hepatologist, and internists were done for evaluation of this persistent severe hypoalbuminemia. Investigations were suggested to exclude inflammatory bowel disease, celiac disease, and other causes of malabsorption, along with Wilson's disease and chronic liver disease.

Urine R/M/E: Protein: +++, red blood cell (RBC) 3–6/high power field (HPF), pus cell 0–2/HPF, 24 hours UTP: 10.1 g/day, UTV: 2,600 mL, serum creatinine: 1.49 mg/day, and serum albumin: 11 g/L.

Following discontinuation of steroid, over the course of 1 year UTP increased to 10 g/day, mycophenolate mofetil 3 g/day was started.

The gastrointestinal survey including stool examination, tissue trans-glutaminase assay, fecal calprotectin, and upper gastrointestinal endoscopy came back normal. Liver function tests (except serum albumin), hepatitis serology, and hepatic ultrasonogram also failed to reveal any abnormalities. However, serum ceruloplasmin was found to be significantly low, along with high urinary copper excretion. A diagnosis of Wilson's disease was made. There were no neurological signs or Kayser–Fleischer ring on slit lamp examination of eye.

Treatment was started with penicillamine and zinc. MMF was continued for another 2 months. But on follow-up, UTP was found to be 15 g/day. At this point, we decided to go for a repeat kidney biopsy. The literature containing associations of Wilson's disease with glomerulonephritis were scarce. The most prevalent was secondary membranous nephropathy due to the use of penicillamine in the treatment process. The other one was immunoglobulin M (IgM) Nephropathy. Repeat kidney biopsy yielded 12 glomeruli. The report left little doubt about focal segmental glomerulosclerosis (FSGS), with focal and segmental sclerosis on light microscopy **(Figs. 1 and 2)**.

There was IgM and C3 deposits on direct immunofluorescence (DIF) study. Having failed with steroid and MMF, we decided to start him on cyclosporine. The initial response was excellent. Within 1 month, UTP came down to 1.5 g/day and serum albumin rose to 30 g/L. He is now on regular follow-up with nephrologists and hepatologists.

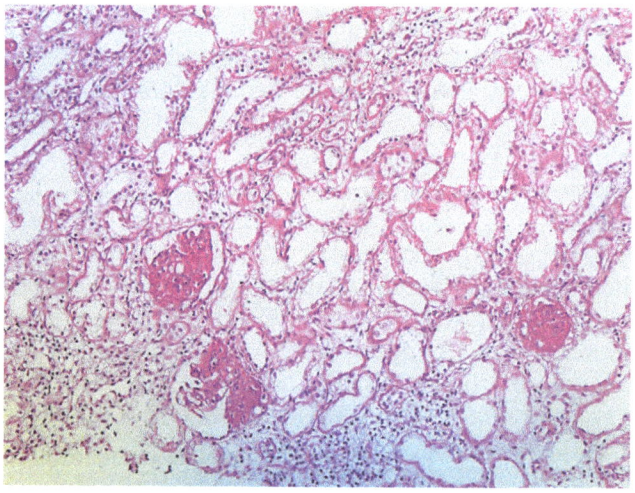

FIG. 1: Focal segmental glomerulosclerosis (FSGS) 10× Periodic acid–Schiff (PAS).

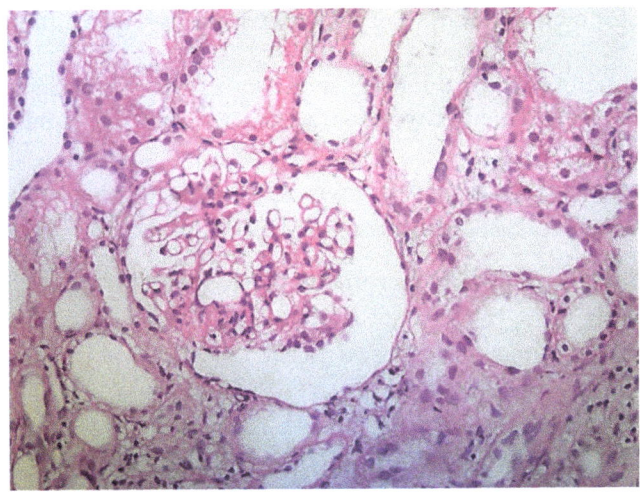

FIG. 2: Focal segmental glomerulosclerosis (FSGS) 20× hematoxylin and eosin (H&E).

■ DISCUSSION

Focal segmental glomerulosclerosis is the most common histological lesion of nephrotic syndrome in adults; about 35% of all cases. It is important to differentiate between primary and secondary FSGS, as the treatment is distinctly different.

Primary FSGS may be related to a circulating factor causing injury to visceral epithelial cells or podocytes.

Secondary FSGS usually results from glomerular hypertrophy and hyperfiltration secondary to infections, drugs, obesity, or previous kidney injury.

Patients with primary FSGS typically present with nephrotic syndrome, while those with secondary FSGS present with non-nephrotic range proteinuria and develop renal insufficiency over time.

We present a case of nephrotic syndrome (FSGS) with Wilson's disease. Wilson's disease is a disorder of copper metabolism due to defective intracellular copper transport in hepatocytes. The mutant gene encodes a copper transporting adenosine triphosphate (ATP) as known as ATP7B, mainly expressed in hepatocytes. It is caused by mutation in the gene encoding the copper transporter ATP7B and hence there is decreases biliary copper excretion and increase hepatic copper accumulation.

Nephrolithiasis may be found in Wilson's patients due to tubular defects in acidification or resultant changes in urinary excretion of substrates that augment stone formation. Wilson's disease may cause acute or severe chronic liver failure leading to hepatorenal syndrome.

Renal injury may occur not only from copper but also from copper-chelating drug, d-penicillamine. Proteinuria of varying degrees may occur even years following initiation of therapy with d-penicillamine in Wilson's disease.

But our patient seems not to be such a case; rather it is case of primary FSGS and Wilson's disease (two separate diseases—a rare coincidence).

FREQUENTLY ASKED QUESTIONS

Q1. What are the morphologic variants of FSGS?

Ans.

- FSGS, not otherwise specified (NOS)
- FSGS, peripheral variant
- FSGS, cellular variant
- FSGS, collapsing variant
- FSGS, tip variant

Q2. What is the prognostic importance of variants of FSGS?

Ans. Outcome is best for tip variant and worst for collapsing variant.

Immunoglobulin M Nephropathy

▪ INTRODUCTION

Mr FK, a 40-year-old nondiabetic businessman, presented to us with a history of generalized swelling and hypertension for 2 years. He was diagnosed as a case of nephrotic syndrome one and a half years back, based on a urinary total protein (UTP) of 3.8 g/day associated with bland urine sediment.

Secondary causes of glomerulonephritis were excluded based on absence of relevant positive clinical features and negative laboratory investigations. He then underwent renal biopsy. Biopsy yielded 21 glomeruli, revealing:

- *Glomerulus*:
  - Size—enlarged
  - Cellularity—proliferation of mesangial cells
  - Matrix—increased
  - Glomerular basement membrane (GBM)—not thick
  - Sclerosis—one segmental, one global
- *Tubules*:
  - Features of protein reabsorption
  - TBM—focally thick
  - Cast—hyaline
- *Interstitium*: Unremarkable
- *Blood vessels*: Unremarkable
- *Direct immunofluorescence (DIF)*:
  - Immunoglobulin M (IgM)
  - Focal segmental deposition
  - Granular pattern
  - 1+
- *Comment*:
  - Mesangial proliferative glomerulonephritis
  - Focal segmental glomerulosclerosis (FSGS)

Correlating these biopsy findings with clinical presentation, a diagnosis of immunoglobulin M nephropathy (IgMN) was made.

He was started on high-dose oral prednisolone (1 mg/kg/day). It was continued for 16 weeks, but he failed to achieve remission. UTP remained at 2.5 g/day at the end of the course and steroid was gradually tapered over a period of 10 weeks. He was then put on mycophenolate mofetil 1.5 g/day for 6 months. This treatment failed to achieve remission as well, UTP remaining at 3.5 g/day. After adequate counseling, oral cyclophosphamide was started at 2 mg/kg/day. It was continued for 4 months, failing to achieve remission. Although he was coprescribed antiproteinuric drugs as well over the course of these 15 months, UTP failed to fall to below 50% of the baseline values, rather went up to 9.7 g/day.

His renal function remained stable (normal) during this period. He was explained that this unremitting proteinuria is a poor prognostic indicator and that most conventional, well-studied treatment options were exhausted. The option of rituximab was presented, since it showed promise in several studies. The cost and side-effects were explained. After dragging around liters of fluid for 2 years, he was quite keen to be an edema-free life and agreed to a course of rituximab.

After excluding possible underlying subclinical infections, 1 g of intravenous (IV) rituximab was administered, followed by another dose of 1 g after 4 weeks. The patient did not appear to have any obvious side-effects with either of the two doses. During the first follow-up after 2 weeks, his proteinuria came down to 2.5 g/day from 9.7 g/day, but went up to 4 g/day before the next dose. After the second dose, his proteinuria again came down to 2 g/day and remained around that level for the next 3 months.

Although he did not achieve complete remission, he was symptomatically improved. We decided to keep him on antiproteinurics and follow-up regularly before deciding on the next course of action.

DISCUSSION

In 1978, two independent research groups led by Cohen et al. and Bhasin et al. reported IgMN in patients who presented with heavy proteinuria and predominant IgM deposition in the mesangial region of glomeruli in a diffuse and global distribution.

The etiology of primary IgMN remains unclear. The glomerular IgM deposits can be seen in some autoimmune and systemic disease. IgMN can affect any age group but mostly involves pediatric and young adult age group. Nephrotic syndrome is the most common clinical finding in pediatric age group; asymptomatic proteinuria and hematuria are common in adults and women, respectively.

Diagnosis of IgMN relies on histopathology. Light microscopic examination reveals minimal or mild mesangial cell proliferation and/or mild mesangial sclerosis. Immunofluorescence is critical in the diagnosis of IgMN and the pattern is a diffuse and global mesangial positivity of IgM with intensity of plus I and greater.

Steroid is the mainstay of treatment with 0–50% resistance. There is little data on the use and response rates of immunosuppressive agents in patients with IgMN. Oral cyclophosphamide has been used with response rate of up to 50%.

Occasional reports show a favorable response to cyclosporine in steroid-dependent IgMN patients. Recurrent disease after renal transplantation has been successfully treated with rituximab in combination with plasma exchange and Igs.

FREQUENTLY ASKED QUESTIONS

Q1. Do IgMN progress to FSGS?

Ans. Yes, about 50% of patients of IgMN could progress to FSGS if unresponsive to corticosteroid.

Q2. What are the variants of minimal change disease (MCD)?

Ans. IgMN and FSGS.

Membranoproliferative Glomerulonephritis

■ INTRODUCTION

Mrs HB, 40 years old, housewife, nondiabetic, newly diagnosed hypertensive, presented with swelling of face and legs along with scanty micturition and dark urine for 10 days. Initially, she noticed swelling around the eyes and face, followed by involvement of the legs. However, swelling was not preceded by fever, sore throat, or any skin infection. She also complains of decreased amount of urine volume, frothy urination, and occasional passage of dark color urine for the same duration. There is no history of chest pain, shortness of breath, cough, jaundice, joint pain, skin rash, oral ulcer, photosensitivity, cold intolerance, or bowel abnormality. She is married for 22 years, mother of three, with no history of miscarriage. Her menstrual period and cycle are normal. Neither there is any significant past history of any disease or hospital admission before this illness nor there is similar sort of illness running in the family. She gives no history of taking herbal or any nephrotoxic medications. She belongs to lower middle class family, lives in a tin-shed house, and is immunized according to Expanded Programme on Immunization (EPI) schedule.

■ ON EXAMINATION

Appearance: Puffy face, anemia: mild, edema: bipedal edema ++, leukonychia: absent, pulse: 84 bpm, blood pressure (BP): 160/90 mm Hg, respiratory rate (RR): 14 breaths/min, jugular venous pressure (JVP): not raised

Temperature: 98°F, lymph nodes: not palpable, thyroid gland: not enlarged, bedside proteinuria +++. Respiratory, cardiovascular, and nervous system examination revealed no abnormality. Fundoscopy was normal.

From history and clinical examination, this seems to be a case of glomerulonephritis with nephritic nephrotic presentation. And it is provisionally diagnosed as a case of membranoproliferative glomerulonephritis (MPGN).

INVESTIGATIONS

- *Urine R/E:* Protein: +++, white blood cell (WBC): 5–6/high power field (HPF), red blood cell (RBC): 10–12/HPF, casts: not found, serum creatinine: 1.2 mg/dL, sodium: 140 mmol/L, potassium: 4.1 mmol/L, chloride: 105 mmol/L, TCO_2: 25.3 mmol/L.
- *Complete blood count (CBC)*: Hemoglobin (Hb): 10 g/dL, erythrocyte sedimentation rate (ESR): 40 mm in 1st hour, mean corpuscular volume (MCV): 69 fl, mean corpuscular hemoglobin (MCH): 28 pg, total count: 7,500/cc, neutrophil: 57%, eosinophil: 4%, lymphocyte: 37%, platelet: 320,000/cc.
- *Serum albumin*: 33 g/dL, urinary total protein (UTP): 2.28 g/day, urinary total volume: 800 mL/day, antinuclear antibody (ANA): negative, antids-DNA: negative, cytoplasmic antineutrophil cytoplasmic antibody (c-ANCA): 1.47 U/L (normal limit), perinuclear antineutrophil cytoplasmic antibody (p-ANCA): 1.22 U/L (normal limit), C3: 0.99 g/L, C4: 0.25 g/L, HBsAg: negative, and antihepatitis C virus (HCV): negative.
- *Total cholesterol*: 156.6 mg/dL, triglyceride: 104.4 mg/dL, high-density lipoprotein (HDL): 21.6 mg/dL, low-density lipoprotein (LDL): 110 mg/dL, fasting blood sugar: 5.1 mmol/L, 2 hours after 75 g glucose: 6.5 mmol/L
- Serum glutamic pyruvic transaminase (SGPT): 21 U/L, thyroid-stimulating hormone (TSH): 2.27 mL/L, urine C/S: no growth, bleeding time: 3 minutes 30 seconds, clotting time: 5 minutes 30 seconds, prothrombin time: 12 seconds, and activated partial thromboplastin time (APTT): 30 seconds
- Ultrasonography of kidney, ureter, and bladder region revealed bipolar diameter of right kidney 9.1 cm, left kidney 9.1 cm, and cortical echogenicity of both kidneys were mildly increased. Corticomedullary differentiations were not well-maintained, pelvicalyceal systems were not dilated.

Renal Biopsy Report (Figs. 1 and 2 and Table 1)

Clinical presentation: Swelling of body for 10 days, urine R/E: albumin: 2+, RBC: plenty, Serum C3: decreased, UTP: 2.28 g/day, serum creatinine: 1.27 mg/dL; nephritic nephrotic presentation.

Gross examination:
- *Received in 10% formalin*: Number of tissue: one, shape: linear, measurement: 1.2 cm

Light microscopic examination (Figs. 1 and 2)
- *Glomerulus*:
  - Number: 14, size: enlarged, lobular accentuation in some glomeruli, cellularity: endocapillary proliferation, matrix: increased (+), glomerular basement membrane (GBM): irregularly thick, additional findings: infiltration of polymorphs.

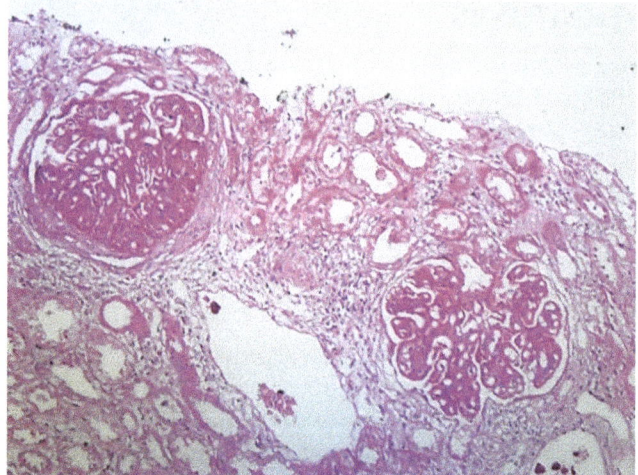

FIG. 1: Membranoproliferative glomerulonephritis Periodic acid-Schiff (PAS).

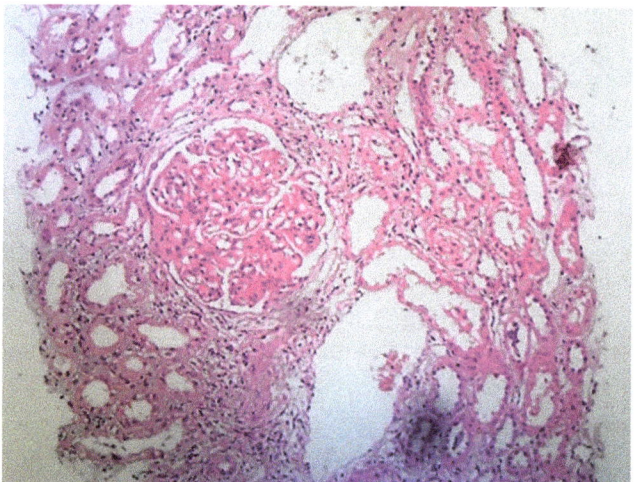

FIG. 2: Membranoproliferative glomerulonephritis hematoxylin and eosin (H&E).

- *Tubule*:
  - *Tubular atrophy*: mild focal, epithelium: features of reabsorption, tuberculous meningitis (TBM): unremarkable, and cast: hyaline.

Interstitium

Inflammation: Focal, chronic inflammatory cells.

Direct Immunofluorescence Finding

Received in 10% normal saline: Number of tissue: one, shape: linear, measurement: 1 cm.

TABLE 1: Direct immunofluorescence (DIF) finding.								
Deposited antibody	IgG	IgM	IgA	C3	Clq	Fibrin	Kappa	Lamda
Site of deposition	Mem+Mes			Mesangium	Mesangium			
Pattern of deposition	Granular			Granular	Granular			
	1+			Trace	1+			

Note: Diagnosis—membranoproliferative glomerulonephritis.

(IgA: immunoglobulin A; IgG: immunoglobulin G; IgM: immunoglobulin M)

DISCUSSION

The case under discussion is one of glomerulonephritis with nephritic presentation with a provisional diagnosis of MPGN.

In fact, MPGN is a histopathologic diagnosis usually causing microscopic hematuria, nephritic nephrotic range proteinuria and renal impairment.

There are two broad categories of MPGN: (1) immune complex mediated and (2) complement mediated (C3 glomerulopathy).

The C3 glomerulopathy; with characteristic bright C3 staining without substantial immunoglobulin deposition is an example of complement mediated MPGN. Dense deposit disease (DDD) with extensive osmiophilic intramembranous sausage-shaped deposition with immunoglobulin staining is attributed to dysregulation of the complement cascade and is in the same spectrum with C3 glomerulopathy. Recognition of this complement-mediated disease must be done by the nephrologist because eculizumab, a monoclonal antibody against terminal products of complement cascade, is a useful therapeutic option in these patients.

The immune complex mediated group can be subdivided by the cause of immune complex formation viz. Infection related (most commonly hepatitis C), monoclonal protein deposition, or an associated autoimmune disease such as systemic lupus erythematosus.

For MPGN with immune complex deposition, treatment targets the source of immune complex production. The three general sources of pathologic immunoglobulin and immune complexes are infection, mono-clonal gammopathy-associated diseases, and autoimmune disorders.

With the identification of hepatitis C, infection is the leading infectious cause of MPGN. Response to antiviral therapy can mitigate the course of the renal disease. A caveat is the occurrence of rapidly progressive glomerulonephritis caused by hepatitis C-associated cryoglobulinemia which requires intense immunosuppression with pulse Solu-medrol followed by high-dose daily steroids, cyclophosphamide, therapeutic apheresis, and the consideration of anti-B-cell therapy in the form of rituximab.

Immune complex deposition formed by monoclonal gammopathy from B-cell dyscrasias responds to immunosuppressive treatment. If criteria are met for multiple myeloma, treatment of the primary disease is indicated, though overt myeloma is usually not the culprit when MGPN with immunoglobulin G (IgG) monoclonal deposits is the diagnosis. If there is evidence of cryoglobulin production and deposition on renal biopsy, then high-dose daily steroids plus cyclophosphamide is indicated. Therapeutic apheresis would be added for rapidly progressive disease as well as the consideration of anti-B-cell therapy in the form of rituximab.

There is a group of patients, where there is no evidence of infection, no monoclonal gammopathy, no systemic autoimmune disease—these are the patients of idiopathic immune complex-mediated MPGN.

In the present case of MPGN, evidence for complement-mediated disease was absent. Working through the differential for a source of the immune complex formation, there was no evidence of infection or monoclonal protein production or deposition; and autoimmune disease is a possible etiology and with extensive subendothelial deposits with multiple immune reactants (IgG, C1q), and given no apparent disease based on history, physical examination, or serologic testing. Thus, we believe, idiopathic immune complex-mediated MPGN is the most accurate diagnosis in our case.

She was clinically stable with stable renal function during the follow-up period. Her proteinuria decreased from 2.28 to 0.5 g/day with treatment with angiotensin-converting enzyme (ACE) inhibitor. Therefore, immediate treatment with conservative therapy (ACE inhibitor) and close follow-up spared her from possible adverse effect of prolonged immunosuppression.

FREQUENTLY ASKED QUESTIONS

Q1. **What are the types of MPGN?**

Ans. Etiologically, MPGN may be idiopathic; may be secondary.

The different histopathological types are:

- *Type I:* Presence of subendothelial deposits of immune complexes associated with activation of the classical complement pathway.
- *Type II (DDD):* Dense deposits within the mesangial and in the basement membranes of the glomeruli, tubules, and Bowman's capsule.
- *Type III:* A variant of type I, extensive subendothelial, and subepithelial electron-dense deposits.

Q2. **What are the common clinical manifestations of MPGN?**

Ans.

- Microscopic hematuria and non-nephrotic proteinuria (35%)
- Nephrotic syndrome with mild renal impairment (35%)
- Chronic kidney disease (CKD) (20%)
- Rapidly deteriorating renal function (10%)

Membranous Nephropathy

■ INTRODUCTION

Mrs SS, 42 years old, housewife, normotensive, nondiabetic, presented with generalized swelling for 3 months. Initially, she noticed swelling around the eyes and face, followed by gradual involvement of the whole body. Swelling was associated with decreased amount of urine volume and frothy but not dark color urine. Moreover it was not preceded by fever, sore throat, or any skin infection. There is no history of chest pain, shortness of breath, cough, jaundice, joint pain, skin rash, oral ulcer, photosensitivity, cold intolerance, bowel disturbance, or weight loss. She is married for 20 years, mother of two, with no history of miscarriage. Her menstrual period and cycle are normal. She had cholecystectomy 2 years back. She gives no history of taking herbal or any nephrotoxic medications. All her family members are in good health. No one has any history of such illness. She belongs to upper middle class family and is immunized according to Expanded Programme on Immunization (EPI) schedule. With the mentioned complaints, she went to a physician who prescribed her diuretics and advised hospitalization for renal biopsy.

■ ON EXAMINATION

Appearance: Puffy face, body built: average, nutrition: average, co-operation: cooperative, decubitus: on choice, anemia: mild, jaundice: absent, edema: bipedal edema (pitting), dehydration: absent, cyanosis: absent, clubbing: absent, koilonychia: absent, leukonychia: absent, pulse: 84 bpm, blood pressure (BP): 130/80 mm Hg, respiratory rate (RR): 14 breaths/min

Jugular venous pressure (JVP): Not raised, temperature: 98°F, lymph nodes: not palpable, thyroid gland: not enlarged, bedside urine examination 3 plus proteinuria

Examination of other systems including fundoscopy reveals no abnormalities.

From history and examination, clinical diagnosis is glomerulonephritis with nephrotic presentation. The differential diagnoses may be membranous nephropathy, focal segmental glomerulosclerosis, adult minimal change disease, mesangial proliferative glomerulonephritis, and lupus nephritis.

CURRENT MEDICATIONS

- Tablet ramipril 2.5 mg   1 + 0 + 0
- Tablet furosemide 40 mg   1 + 1 + 0
- Tablet atorvastatin 20 mg   0 + 0 + 1
- Tablet famotidine 20 mg   1 + 0 + 1 (before meal)
- Modified ponticelli regimen

INVESTIGATIONS

- *Urine R/E:* Protein: +++, pus cell: 1– 2/high power field (HPF), red blood cell (RBC): 3–4/HPF, casts: not found, urinary total protein (UTP): 7.236 g/day, 24 hours urinary total volume: 1,200 mL, serum albumin: 2.5 g/dL, serum creatinine: 0.93 mg/dL, sodium: 140 mmol/L, potassium: 4.1 mmol/L, chloride: 101 mmol/L, and TCO_2: 25 mmol/L
- *Urine C/S:* No growth
- *Complete blood count (CBC):* Hemoglobin (Hb): 9.8 g/dL, erythrocyte sedimentation rate (ESR): 50 mm in 1st hour, total count: 6,500/cc, neutrophil: 55%, eosinophil: 2%, lymphocyte: 29%, platelet: 370,000/cc
- *Antinuclear antibody (ANA):* Negative, anti-ds-DNA: negative, cytoplasmic antineutrophil cytoplasmic antibodies (c-ANCA): 1.54 U/L (normal limit), perinuclear antineutrophil cytoplasmic antibody (p-ANCA): 1.30 U/L (normal limit), C3: 1.4 g/L (normal), C4: 0.4 g/L (normal), HBsAg: negative, antihepatitis C virus antibody (HCV): negative, total cholesterol: 359 mg/dL, triglyceride: 972 mg/dL, high-density lipoprotein (HDL): 33 mg/dL, low-density lipoprotein (LDL): 150 mg/dL, fasting blood sugar: 5.4 mmol/L, 2 hours after 75 g glucose: 6.3 mmol/L, serum glutamic pyruvic transaminase (SGPT): 21 U/L, thyroid-stimulating hormone (TSH): 2.17 mIU/L
- *Antiphospholipase A2 receptor (PLA2R) antibody:* Positive
- Bleeding time: 3 minutes 30 seconds, clotting time: 5 minutes 30 seconds, prothrombin time: 14 seconds, activated partial thromboplastin time (APTT): 30 seconds

Ultrasonographic of Kidney, Ureter, and Bladder Region

- *Kidneys:* Right kidney 10.5 cm, left kidney 10.8 cm, cortical echogenicity both kidneys are normal, corticomedullary differentiation (CMD) is maintained, pelvicalyceal systems are not dilated.
- *Chest X-ray posteroanterior (P/A) view:* Normal study

Renal Biopsy Report (Figs. 1 and 2 and Table 1)

Light Microscopic Examination (Figs. 1 and 2)

- *Glomerulus*: Number: 20, size: enlarged, cellularity: not increased, matrix: increased, glomerular basement membrane (GBM): thick. sclerosis: 1 global (1/20), crescent: absent, K-W bodies: absent, fibrin cap: absent, and capsular drop: absent.

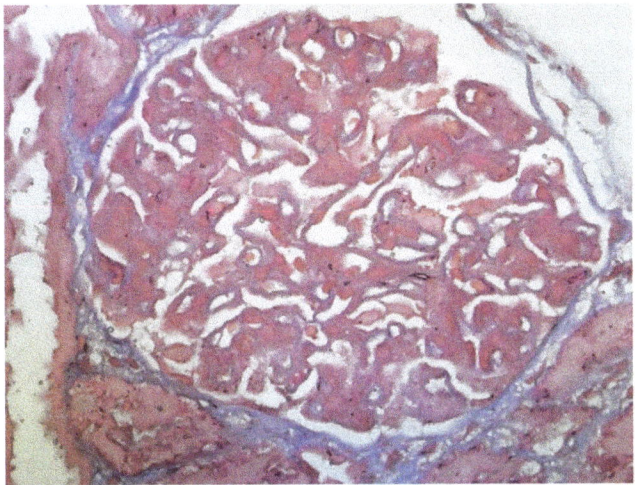

FIG. 1: Membranous nephropathy [Periodic acid–Schiff (PAS) is a staining] 40× magnification.

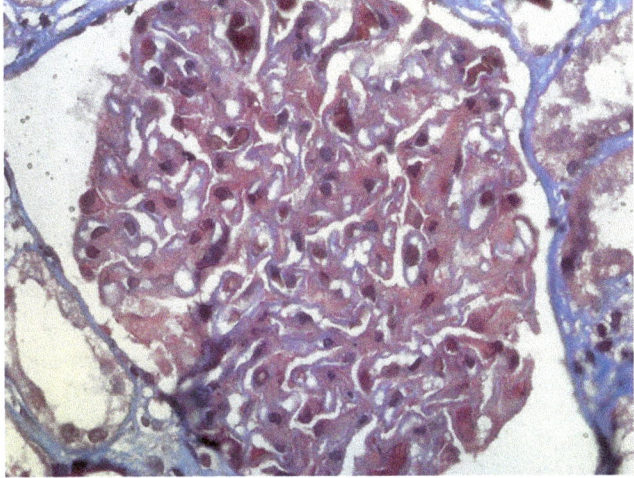

FIG. 2: Membranous nephropathy silver stain 40× magnification.

TABLE 1: Direct immunofluorescence (DIF) findings.								
Deposited antibody	**IgG**	**IgA**	**IgM**	**C3**	**C1q**	**Fibrin**	**Kappa**	**Lamda**
Site of deposition	MEM			MEM			MEM	MEM
Pattern of deposition	Granular			Granular			Granular	Granular
Intensity	3+			1+			2+	1+

(IgA: immunoglobulin A; IgG: immunoglobulin G; IgM: immunoglobulin M)

- *Tubule*:
  - T. atrophy—focal
  - Epithelium—features of protein reabsorption.
  - Tubular basement membrane (TBM)—thick
- *Interstitium*:
  - *Inflammation*: Mild and chronic

DIAGNOSIS

Membranous nephropathy

DISCUSSION

Our patient, 42 years of age, female, presented with nephrotic syndrome. Renal biopsy was done and a diagnosis of membranous nephropathy was made. She had positive anti-PLA2R antibody.

She was put on angiotensin-converting enzyme inhibitor (ACEI), atorvastatin, and a combination of daily oral dose of cyclophosphamide 2 mg/kg/day alternating monthly with corticosteroids (methylprednisolone pulses 3 × 1 g intravenously at months 1, 3, and 5 and oral prednisolone 0.5 mg/kg alternate days for 6 months.

Her proteinuria decreased from 7.2 g/day to 750 mg/day at the end of the 6-month course.

FREQUENTLY ASKED QUESTIONS

Q1. Is spontaneous remission possible in membranous nephropathy?

Ans. Spontaneous remission in proteinuria has been reported in up to 30% cases. Female gender and non-nephrotic proteinuria at presentation are the features associated with spontaneous remission.

Q2. **What are the indication of disease-specific treatment in membranous nephropathy?**

Ans.

- Proteinuria >4 g/day with no decrease >50% after 6 months ACEI/ angiotensin receptor blocker (ARB)
- Proteinuria >8 g/day for 6 months
- Life-threatening complication of nephrotic syndrome
- Rapid deterioration of kidney function not otherwise explained
- PLA2R antibody >150 RU/mL

Henoch–Schönlein Purpura Nephritis

■ INTRODUCTION

Md I, 20 years old student, normotensive, nondiabetic hailing from Keraniganj, Dhaka, presented with the complaints of rash on both lower limbs for 2 months, swelling of face and lower limbs along with dark color urine for same duration. Rash is present for 2 months involving up to both knees, which is palpable, non-itchy, with no discharge. He also noticed swelling around the eyes and face, followed by involvement of the legs for last 2 months. However, swelling was not preceded by fever, sore throat, or any skin infection. He complains of passage of dark color urine for the same duration which is not associated with burning sensation during micturition, or loin pain. There is no history of chest pain, shortness of breath, cough, jaundice, oral ulcer, photosensitivity, abdominal pain, arthralgia, or bloody diarrhea. At the age of 13 years, he suffered from similar sort of swelling, dark color, and frothy urine along with renal impairment. At that time he was treated with corticosteroid (prednisolone 1 mg/kg/day) for 8 weeks which was tapered over 6 months. He was in drug-free remission for 7 years. There is no similar sort of illness running in the family. He gives no history of taking herbal or any nephrotoxic medications. He belongs to lower middle class family and is immunized according to Expanded Programme on Immunization (EPI) schedule.

■ ON EXAMINATION

Patient is conscious, oriented, and co-operative, anemia: absent, nonicteric, weight: 67 kg, pulse: 70 bpm, regular blood pressure (BP): 100/70 mm Hg, temperature: 98.2°F, respiratory rate: 18 breaths/min, no lymphadenopathy, thyroid gland: not enlarged, jugular venous pressure (JVP): not raised, edema: bilateral pitting pedal edema present, skin condition: palpable purpuric rash on both lower limbs (**Fig. 1**), and bedside urine dipstick reveals +++ proteinuria.

Systemic examination including fundoscopy reveals no abnormalities. From history and clinical examination,

The provisional diagnosis may be immunoglobulin A (IgA) vasculitis.

INVESTIGATIONS

- *Urine R/E*: Urine was dark red **(Fig. 2)**, protein: +++, red blood cell (RBC): plenty, pus cell: 3–5/high power field (HPF), cast: nil.
- Urinary total protein (UTP) and urinary total volume (UTV): UTP: 4.1 g/day, UTV: 2,600 mL/day

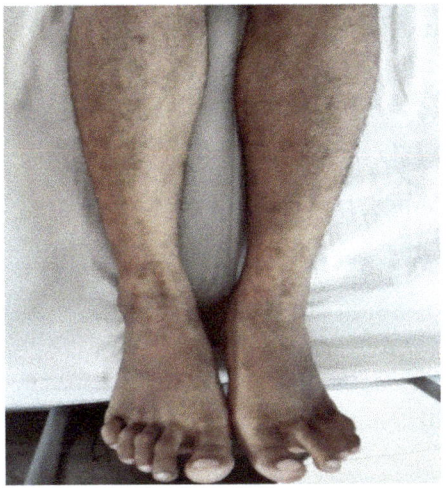

FIG. 1: Rash over extensor surface of lower limb.

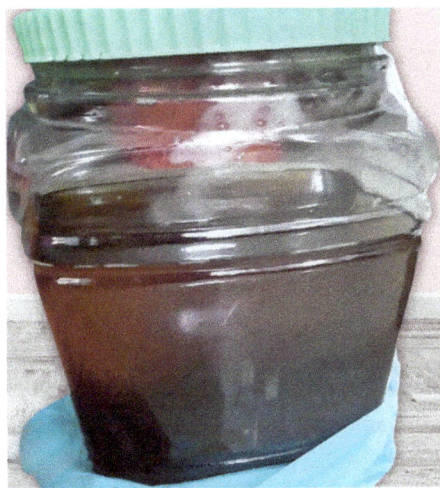

FIG. 2: Dark red color urine.

- *Serum urea and serum creatinine*: Serum creatinine (0.6–1.3 mg/dL): 1.9 mg/dL, serum urea (10–50 mg/dL) (1.8–7.2 mmol/L): 61 mg/dL
- *Serum electrolytes*: Sodium (Na^+): 137.8 mmol/L, potassium (K^+): 5.0 mmol/L, chloride (Cl): 102.3 mmol/L, CO_2: 25.0 mmol/L
- *Complete blood count (CBC)*: Hemoglobin (Hb): 12.8 g/dL, erythrocyte sedimentation rate (ESR): 70 mm in 1st hour, WBC: 11.50 × 10^9/L, platelet: 720 × 10^9/L, WBC: 4.74 × 10^{12}/L
- *Others*: Perinuclear antineutrophil cytoplasmic antibody (p-ANCA): negative, cytoplasmic antineutrophil cytoplasmic antibodies (c-ANCA): negative, antinuclear antibody (ANA): negative, C3 (80–170 mg/dL): 132 mg/dL, C4 (20–50 mg/dL): 32 mg/dL, albumin (38–50 g/L): 27.3 g/L, bleeding time (BT): 2 minutes 30 seconds, CT: 5 minutes 45 seconds, and prothrombin time (PT): 15.20 seconds

Ultrasonography of Kidney, Ureter, and Bladder (Fig. 3)

- Both the kidneys are swollen.
- Right kidney measures about 10.9 × 5.1 cm and left kidney measures about 11.2 × 6.7 cm.
- Cortical echogenicity is increased. Corticomedullary differentiation is reduced.
- Pelvicalyceal systems are not dilated.
- Urinary bladder is well-filled and appears normal.
- Prostate is normal in size with uniform echotexture.

Impression: Bilateral acute renal parenchymal disease.

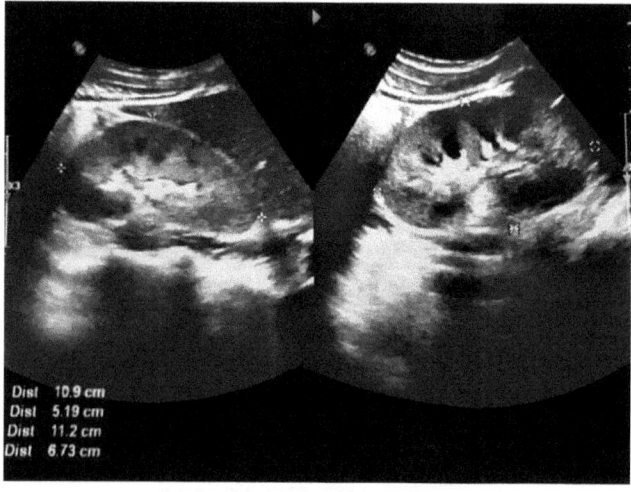

Dist   10.9 cm
Dist   5.19 cm
Dist   11.2 cm
Dist   6.73 cm

FIG. 3: Ultrasonography (USG) of kidney, ureter, and bladder (KUB) region.

SKIN BIOPSY REPORT

- *Microscopic appearance*: Sections show skin. The epidermis reveals mild hyperkeratosis. The upper dermis shows infiltration of chronic inflammatory cells in and around the blood vessels. Few extravasated RBC is also seen.
- *Direct immunofluorescence (DIF) findings*: Cryostat sections of skin do not show any deposition of immunoglobulin G (IgG), immunoglobulin M (IgM), IgA, C3, and fibrinogen.
- *Diagnosis*: Small vessel vasculitis

RENAL BIOPSY REPORT

Refer to **Tables 1 and 2**.

TABLE 1: Light microscopy.			
Received in 10% formalin			
Glomerulus	Number	16	Crescent: Cellular (4/16)
	Size	Enlarged	
	Cellularity	Proliferation of endocapillary and mesangial cells	
	Matrix	Increased	
	GBM	Mildly thick	
	Additional findings	Inflammatory cells with nuclear debris	
Tubule	Epithelium	Features of protein reabsorption	Tubulitis: Present Others: Focal tubular injury
	Cast	RBC, hyaline	
Inflammation	Chronic inflammatory cells including eosinophils		Edema
Blood vessels	Thick-walled	Mildly thick	*Vasculitis*: Mild features of vasculitis

(GBM: glomerular basement membrane; RBC: red blood cell)

TABLE 2: Direct immunofluorescence (DIF) finding (Received in normal saline).						
Deposited antibody	IgG	IgM	IgA	C3	C1q	Fibrin
Site of deposition	GBM		Mesangium	Mes + Blood Vessels	Mesangium	
Pattern of deposition	Linear		Granular	Granular	Granular	
Intensity	1+		1+	2+	1+	

DIAGNOSIS

- Henoch–Schönlein purpura (HSP) nephritis
- Infection-associated glomerulonephritis (GN)
- Lupus nephritis

DISCUSSION

Henoch–Schönlein purpura nephritis is a leukocytoclastic vasculitis primarily seen in children, with involvement of skin, joints by nonthrombocytopenic palpable purpura, arthritis, and gastrointestinal (GI) and renal involvement. The etiology of the disease is not clear. In HSP, cutaneous involvement is the most common presentation. Purpuric skin lesions are typically localized in the lower extremities, as in the present case. But rash may also be seen in hip, hands, and arms.

Renal involvement in adult with HSP is not different from IgA nephropathy. Tissue confirmation of IgA deposition by renal or skin biopsy is necessary to establish the diagnosis. Much of the renal involvement in HSP is transient. Urine abnormalities are noted during the acute presentation but may disappear. Asymptomatic urine abnormalities is most common. Nephrotic syndrome occurs in 20–30% of patients. Acute kidney injury (AKI) may also develop as a result of crescentic GN. Our patient had raised serum creatinine at presentation which resolved with treatment but there was no crescent formation at the time when renal biopsy was done. Immunofluorescent microscopy showed granular deposition of IgA and C3 in the mesangium skin biopsy showed infiltration of chronic inflammatory cells in and around blood vessels. But there was no deposition of IgA.

The treatment of IgAN with proteinuria of >1 g/24 hours remains controversial. Tight control of BP and proteinuria with angiotensin-converting enzyme (ACE) inhibitors and angiotensin-receptor blocker (ARB) should be first line of treatment. Corticosteroids should be considered only if proteinuria above 1 g/24 hours persists on maximal ACE inhibitor or ARB therapy.

FREQUENTLY ASKED QUESTIONS

Q1. What is the usual distribution of rash in HSP?

Ans. Mainly on the extensor surfaces of legs, feet, and buttock. Can also appear on arms, face, and trunk; may be worse on areas of pressure such as the sock line and waistline. The rash does not blanch on pressure.

Q2. **What are the indications of specific treatment (steroid) in HSP?**

Ans. Indications of steroid are:

- Persistent nephrotic syndrome
- Crescents in >50% of glomeruli
- Severe abdominal pain
- Substantial GI hemorrhage
- Severe soft tissue edema
- Severe scrotal edema
- Neurological involvement

  Plasmapheresis or high-dose intravenous immunoglobulin (IVIg) may be recommended for worsening renal function hemorrhage in lung and brain refractory to steroid and immunosuppressive drugs.

Alport Syndrome

▮ INTRODUCTION

Mr AT, 25-year-old student, hypertensive for 9 months, nondiabetic, presented with the complaints of progressive decline in renal function for 9 months. He was reasonably well 9 months back. At that time, he developed anorexia, nausea, and weakness. During evaluation, he was found to have renal impairment (serum creatinine: 5.96 mg/dL). A diagnosis of chronic kidney disease was made and he was put on conservative management.

His renal function was stable till July 2021. For the last 2 months, his renal function is progressively worsening. It was not associated with puffiness of face, reduction in urine volume, passage of high color urine, burning sensation during micturition, or dysuria. There is no history of volume loss, fever, loin pain, skin rash, arthralgia, nephrotoxic medication or drug abuse, jaundice, or liver disease. He does however give history of taking traditional herbal remedies preceding this illness.

He gives history of deafness in both ears noticed at the age of 12 years, gradually progressive, not associated with earache, discharge, or tinnitus. He also complains of gradual dimness of vision for 2 months in both eyes, but no pain, redness, or discharge.

Among the three siblings, two of his elder brothers died before the age of 30 years. Both of them had severe renal failure and needed hemodialysis. Both had deafness. Neither his sister (20 years old) nor his parents have renal disease. No history of consanguineous marriage in his family. He is immunized as per Expanded Programme on Immunization (EPI) schedule but not vaccinated against hepatitis B virus (HBV), *Influenzae*, or *Pneumococcus*.

Examination revealed puffy face, pedal edema, and a bedside urine dipstick showing ++ proteinuria. Weber test showed no lateralization and Rinne test was positive in both ears. Visual acuity was diminished for distant vision. Ophthalmologic along with other relevant examinations revealed normal findings.

A provisional diagnosis of Alport syndrome (AS) is made.

▌ INVESTIGATIONS

Renal function test and complete blood count **(Table 1)**.

TABLE 1: Renal function test and complete blood count (CBC).	
Serum creatinine	9.2 mg/dL
Na$^+$	140
K$^+$	3.4
Cl$^-$	104
TCO$_2$	27
Hb%	9.8 g/dL
ESR	20 (mm/1st hour)
WBC	11,000/µL
N	87%
Platelet count	200,000/µL

(ESR: erythrocyte sedimentation rate; Hb: hemoglobin; WBC: white blood cell)

Other Laboratory Parameters

- *24 hours urinary total protein (UTP)*: 3.6 g/day
- *Ferritin*: 71.87 ng/mL
- *Transferrin saturation (TSAT)*: 37%
- *Serum albumin*: 30 g/L
- *Serum calcium*: 8.0 mg/dL
- *Serum phosphate*: 3.1 mg/dL
- *Serum uric acid*: 6.5 mg/dL
- *Intact parathyroid hormone (iPTH)*: 84.6 pg/mL
- *Random blood sugar (RBS)*: 5.3 mmol/L
- *Thyroid-stimulating hormone (TSH)*: 3.83 uIU/mL
- *Antinuclear antibody (ANA)*: Negative
- *Perinuclear antineutrophil cytoplasmic antibody (p-ANCA) and cytoplasmic antineutrophil cytoplasmic antibodies (c-ANCA)*: Negative
- *C3 and C4*: Normal
- *HBsAg*: Negative
- *Antihepatitis C virus (HCV)*: Negative
- Ultrasonography of kidney, ureter, and bladder:
  - Bipolar length of right kidney is 8.1 cm and left kidney is 8.0 cm.
  - Cortical echogenicity is increased.
  - Corticomedullary differentiation (CMD) is lost.
  - *Comment*: Bilateral renal parenchymal disease

- *Audiological report*: Bilateral moderate-to-severe sensorineural type of hearing loss
- *Fundoscopic examination*: (by indirect ophthalmoscope)—
  ○ Maculopathy on B/E (Lt>Rt)
  ○ B/L perimacular flecks
  ○ Features of exudative retinal detachment on left eye
- *Slit-lamp examination*: No anterior lenticonus
  He was put on maintenance hemodialysis.

■ DISCUSSION

Alport syndrome is an inherited disorder of the basement membranes due to mutations affecting specific proteins of the type IV collagen family. The usual presentation of AS includes hematuria, proteinuria and declining renal function, sensorineural deafness, and ocular abnormalities. Affected males usually have severe form of disease and in females the disease is usually mild. Three forms of AS have been recognized based on molecular genetics. Alport syndrome results from mutations in the *COL4A5* (X-linked) or *COL4A3/COL4A4* (recessive) genes. An X-linked AS is the predominant form of the disease (80%). Male patients with this form of disease progress to end-stage renal disease (ESRD) during the second or third decade of life and have deafness. Autosomal recessive AS presents with typical clinical and pathologic features of disease but lacks a positive family history. Most patients with this form develop ESRD and deafness before 30 years of age. Autosomal dominant forms of disease present with asymptomatic hematuria and have a slower course to ESRD.

There are no pathognomonic lesions by light microscopy or direct immunofluorescence in AS. Electron microscopy reveals diagnostic abnormalities. The cardinal structural features are variable thickening, thinning, basket weaving, and lamellation of glomerular basement membrane (GBM). Absence of α3, α4, α5 chains of type IV collagen from GBM and distal tubular basement membrane is a diagnostic finding.

Renal transplantation is the only available treatment. Graft survival is equivalent to other primary diagnosis. However, anti-GBM glomerulonephritis involving the graft is rare (2–3% in male patients).

FREQUENTLY ASKED QUESTIONS

Q1. Is there any role of drug treatment in AS?

Ans. Cyclosporine appeared to stabilize renal function in a small uncontrolled study. Angiotensin-converting enzyme (ACE) inhibitors may have some beneficial effect in retarding progression to ESRD.

Q2. Is renal transplantation contraindicated in AS?

Ans. Renal transplantation is not contraindicated in AS. However, anti-GBM glomerulonephritis involving the renal allograft may occur in 2–3% patients.

Lipomyelomeningocele with Tethered Cord Syndrome, Neurogenic Bladder, CKD, and Disseminated Tuberculosis

▌ INTRODUCTION

Mr B, a 38-year-old nondiabetic, normotensive, a known case of chronic kidney disease (CKD), presented to us with epistaxis and deteriorating renal function for 2 months.

According to the patient's mother, since the age of 5 years, he had frequent urinary and fecal incontinence. At 10 years of age following a motor bike accident, he developed lower limb weakness and worsening of urinary incontinence. After a year, although his weakness improved, urinary incontinence persisted. At the 18 years of age, he consulted for his problem and was advised to do clean intermittent self-catheterization (CISC) but refused to do so and was trying to lead a normal life. However, he could not control his symptoms and needed frequent hospital and doctor visits. At 27 years of age, during further evaluation, he was diagnosed to have neurogenic bladder with urinary tract infection (UTI) and was again advised to do CISC, which he did on irregular basis up to 34 years of age.

But at this time, his symptoms exaggerated, for which he underwent extensive evaluation. His left kidney was found to be nonfunctioning according to ^{99m}Tc-diethylenetriaminepentaacetate (DTPA) renogram along with hydronephrosis. He was advised for left-sided nephrectomy, but denied to do so. At that time after neurological consultation, he was also diagnosed as a case of lipomyelomeningocele with tethered cord syndrome for which further evaluation was suggested but he refused.

At 36 years of age, urodynamic study revealed acontractile bladder.

Since then he had several episodes of UTI and one episode of acute kidney injury (AKI).

For last 5 months, he developed low-grade fever, anorexia, weight loss, macroscopic hematuria, cough, abdominal heaviness, and was diagnosed as a case of disseminated tuberculosis (TB) (with involvement of kidney, spleen, liver, lungs, L1 vertebra, and abdominal lymph nodes). At the same time, he was also diagnosed as idiopathic thrombocytopenic purpura (ITP).

Anti-TB was started as following (adjusted according to weight and renal function):

- Tablet rimactazid 300 mg (2 + 0 + 0) to continue for 6 months
- Tablet pyrazinamide 500 mg (3 + 0 + 0) for 2 months
- Tablet ethambutol 400 mg (1 + 0 + 0) for 2 months
- Tablet eltrombopag (thrombopoietin receptor agonist) 25 mg was given for management of ITP.

After 20 days of getting anti-TB medications, his renal function further deteriorated and at this time, he developed right-sided hydronephrosis.

Double J (DJ) stenting was done in the right side. Approximately 1 month after placement DJ stent was displaced and it was repositioned. Foley's urinary catheterization was done at the same setting.

However, he was referred from urology to nephrology department as his renal function was further deteriorating.

He had epistaxis of fresh blood, two to three times in a day, 2–3 mL in each episode for 2 months and hematology referral was given and they advised:

- Tablet ETP (50 mg) 1 + 0 + 0
- Pulse Dexa (40 mg) 1 + 0 + 0.....D1–D4
- Platelet concentrate

He also had an injury of great toe of left foot and developed cellulitis.

List of medications:

- Injection imipenem 500 mg IV 12 hourly
- Capsule flucloxacillin 500 mg 1 + 1 + 1 + 1
- Tablet rimactazid 300 mg 2 + 0 + 0
- Tablet ETP 50 mg 1 + 0 + 0
- Tablet calbo 500 mg 1 + 0 + 1
- Tablet febuxostat 40 mg 0 + 0 + 1

ON EXAMINATION

- *Body built*: Average
- *Weight*: 57 kg
- Clawing of toes present **(Fig. 1)**
- There is a nontender, soft, swelling measuring about 3 × 2 cm in diameter located at lumbosacral region.

Bedside urine heat coagulation test:
Protein: Nil

SYSTEMIC EXAMINATION

Detected no abnormality.

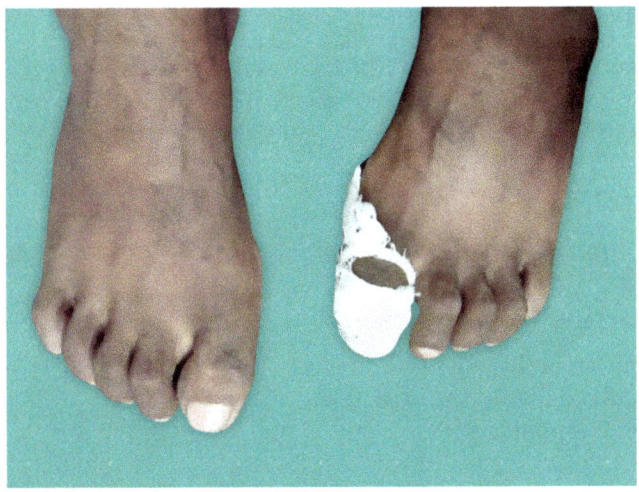

FIG. 1: Clawing of toes.

◼ INVESTIGATIONS (TABLE 1 AND OTHER LABORATORY PARAMETERS)

Urine R/M/E: Albumin + +, white blood cell (WBC)—plenty, red blood cell (RBC) plenty, and no cast

Urine C/S: Growth of *Candida*

Urinary total protein 3 g/day

Serum creatinine: 5.46 mg/dL

Serum electrolytes: Na^+ 134, K^+ 3.5, Cl—100

TABLE 1: Other biochemical tests.	
Serum urea	55 mg/dL
Serum uric acid	9 mg/dL
Serum calcium	8.9 mg/dL
Serum phosphate	6.8 mg/dL
IPTH	378/L
Serum albumin	3.1 g/L
Serum iron	3.3 µmol/L
Serum ferritin	1742 ng/mL
TIBC	27 µmol/L
CRP	122 mg/dL

(CRP: C-reactive protein; iPTH: intact parathyroid hormone; TIBC: total iron-binding capacity)

Complete Blood Count

Hemoglobin (Hb) 9.2 g/dL, erythrocyte sedimentation rate (ESR) 83 mm in 1st hour, total count white blood cell (TC WBC) 12,000/mm^3, N: 83%, L—11%, m—3%, E—3%, and platelet court 500,000/cmm.

Peripheral Blood Film

Anemia of chronic disease with lymphopenia and thrombocytopenia.

Bone Marrow Examination

- Secondary reactive change
- Peripheral consumption of platelet
- Erythroid hypoplasia

Chest X-ray Posteroanterior View (Fig. 2)

Computed Tomography (CT) of Kidneys, Ureters and Bladder (KUB)

Clinical information: For evaluation of right renal mass.

Technique: Pre- and postcontrast multislice computerized tomography (CT) of kidneys, ureters and bladder (KUB) was performed.

Findings

Right kidney: Nephrogram and pyelogram are prompt. Mild heterogeneously enhancing mixed density lesion with calcification within is noted in lower

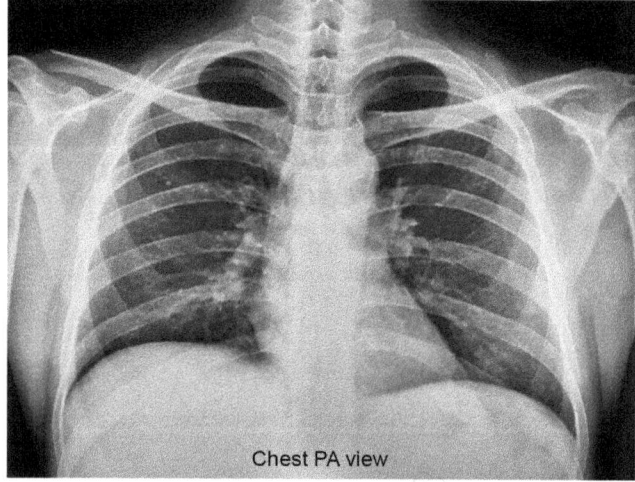

Chest PA view

FIG. 2: Miliary lung lesion. Diffuse miliary densities are seen in both lungs fields.

pole region of right kidney measuring about 5.0 × 5.4 cm. Small stones are seen in mid and lower calyx. Small cyst is noted in upper pole. Hypodense area measuring about 2.1 × 1.5 cm is noted in upper pole region. Anterior lower calyx is distorted. Rests of calyces are mildly dilated. Right lower ureter is beaded in appearance.

Left kidney: No nephrogram and pyelogram are seen. It is irregular in contour. Multiple hypodense lesions are seen in left kidney.

Adrenal gland: The adrenal glands are unremarkable.

Urinary bladder: The urinary bladder is partially filled. Bladder base is irregular.

Balloon of Foley catheter is seen in situ.

Prostate: Normal in size with homogeneous tissue density. Capsule appears intact.

No ascites or abdominal lymphadenopathy are detected.

Lytic lesion is seen in L1 vertebral body. Spinal dysraphism is noted in sacral region.

Spleen in mildly enlarged in size and shows diffuse small hypodense lesions.

Liver is enlarged in size.

Enlarged para-aortic and mesenteric lymph nodes are detected.

Impression
- Overall CT features suggest disseminated tuberculosis involving the kidneys, spleen, lungs, L1 vertebra, and abdominal lymph nodes.
- Right renal calculi
- Nonexcreting left kidney-associated multiple abscesses
- Spinal dysraphism in sacral region

■ DISCUSSION

Lipomyelomeningocele is a condition where spinal cord will have fat at the lower tip and this fat may connect to the fat that overlies the thecal sac and this leads to tethering of spinal cord. Tethered spinal cord syndrome is a neurological disorder caused by tissue attachments that limit the movement of the spinal cord within the spinal column. This attachment causes an abnormal stretching of the spinal cord. Loss of bladder and bowel control is one of the features due to increasing sensory and motor deficits caused by strain on the spinal cord as in our patient. This patient had neurogenic bladder and obstructive uropathy leading to CKD.

The leading urological causes of CKD include obstructive uropathy, reflux nephropathy, and kidney aplasia/hypoplasia/dysplasia. Obstructive uropathy and aplastic/hypoplastic/dysplastic kidneys each account for 16% of patients in the NAPRCT (North American Pediatric Renal Trials and Collaborative study) registry.

Diagnosis of the tethered cord syndrome is made by history, clinical presentation, and some investigations such as magnetic resonance imaging (MRI), computed tomography (CT) scan or myelogram. Disseminated tuberculosis (a separate disease perhaps due to compromised immune system) is a mycobacterial infection in which *Mycobacteria* have spread from the lungs to other parts of the body through blood or lymph system.

FREQUENTLY ASKED QUESTIONS

Q1. How common are urologic causes of CKD?

Ans. Data obtained from CKD in children (CKiD) cohort study underlying urological causes of CKD were present in 59% children.

Q2. What is the duration of anti-TB treatment in disseminated TB?

Ans. The duration may be 6–12 months depending on the patient condition and choice of the treating physician.

Q3. Is neurogenic bladder a contraindication to renal transplantation?

Ans. Renal transplantation in patients with abnormal lower urinary tract is safe and effective. Patients with ileal conduits do well and have few substantial difficulties. However, preoperative assessment of bladder emptying and urodynamics are important in these patients.

Systemic Lupus Erythematous, Lupus Nephritis, and Avascular Necrosis of Femoral Head

◼ INTRODUCTION

Mrs FA, 34-year-old housewife, hypertensive, nondiabetic presented with bilateral leg swelling for 2 years and pain in both hip joints for 1 year. The swelling was associated with excessive hair loss and oral ulcer, but no skin rash or no joint pain. At that time, she was found to have proteinuria of 2.43 g/day. Although antinuclear antibody (ANA) and antids-DNA were negative. No renal biopsy was performed. Rather treatment was started empirically with oral cyclophosphamide 100 mg/day for 2 months along with high-dose oral prednisolone which was tapered over 1 year. With this treatment, her symptoms subsided. She was not on regular follow-up, during the tapering phase of her steroid, she developed noninflammatory pain in both hip joints, which increased during walking.

She came this time for further evaluation of her illness. She was found to have positive ANA, antids-DNA, low C3 and C4, positive perinuclear antineutrophil cytoplasmic antibody (p-ANCA) with urine protein/creatinine ratio (UPCR) of 4.13 mg/g. Her serum creatinine was increased to 3.4 from 1.7 mg/dL. We performed renal biopsy. Biopsy yielded six glomeruli, revealing:

- *Glomerulus*:
  - Endocapillary proliferation with lobular accentuation
  - Wire loop lesion
  - Double contour of glomerular capillary wall
  - One globally sclerosed
  - One cellular crescent with necrotizing change
- *Tubules*:
  - Acute tubular injury with red cell cast
  - Tubular atrophy

- *Interstitium*:
    ○ Focal lymphocytic infiltration
    ○ Interstitial fibrosis
- *Blood vessel*: Unremarkable

Direct immunofluorescence (DIF): Full house deposition of complements and immunoglobulins in granular pattern along glomerular basement membrane (GBM) and mesangium.

Comment: Diffuse proliferative lupus nephritis (LN), International Society of Nephrology (ISN)/Renal Pathology Society (RPS) LN class IV, G (A).

For evaluation of hip pain, we performed a series of imaging, which revealed:
- *X-ray of hip joint (Figs. 1 and 2)*:
    ○ Crescentic lucency with sclerosis in subarticular region of both femoral head (more on left side)
    ○ Minimal collapse of left femoral head
    Comment: Suggestive of avascular necrosis (AVN) of both femoral head (more on left) with early collapse of left head.
- *Magnetic resonance imaging (MRI) of hip joints*:
    ○ AVN of both femoral head, prominent on left side. Ficat stage II

Correlating these investigation findings with clinical presentation, a diagnosis of class IV LN with AVN of both femur bone head (Lt > Rt) was made.

She was started with intravenous (IV) methylprednisolone 1 g daily for three consecutive days, followed by oral prednisolone 1 mg/kg/day along with mycophenolate Na 720 mg twice daily. With this treatment, she achieved remission within 2 weeks. Serum creatinine came down to 1.4 mg/day and 24 hours urinary total protein (UTP) to 0.4 g/day. High-dose oral prednisolone was continued for 1 month and then gradually tapered

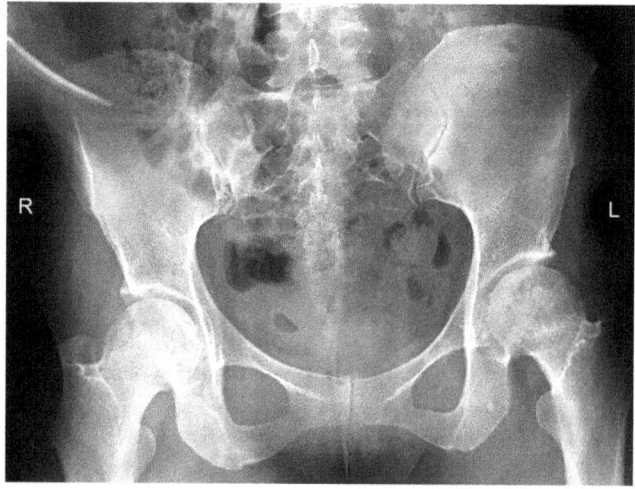

FIG. 1: X-ray of hip joints anteroposterior (AP) view.

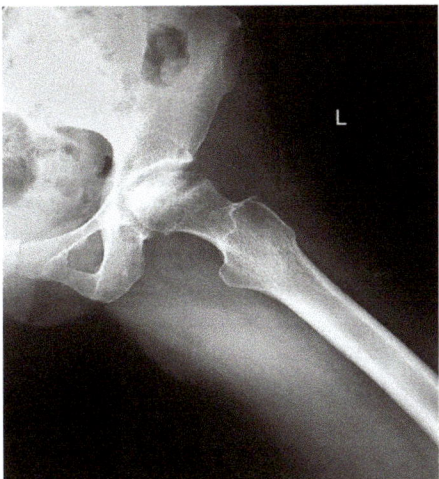

FIG. 2: X-ray of left hip joint.

off to 7.5 mg/day. Hypertension was well-controlled with telmisartan 80 mg once daily and amlodipine 5 mg once daily.

Regarding AVN, orthopedic consultation was taken and decision was taken to keep her on conservative management with a plan to go for total hip replacement in case of further deterioration.

■ DISCUSSION

The incidence and prevalence of LN are influenced by age, gender, ethnicity, geographic region, and diagnostic criteria employed. The peak incidence of lupus is 15–45 years with female preponderance (10:1). The gender predominance is less in children and older people. Among lupus patients, LN affects both male and female equally but prognostically bad in children and men.

About 30–50% of systemic lupus erythematous (SLE) patients will have clinically evident renal disease at presentation. During follow-up, about 60% adult patients develop renal disease. Renal involvement is manifested by proteinuria, active urinary sediment with microhematuria, dysmorphic red blood cell (RBC) and RBC cast in urine, and hypertension. Sometimes, a renal involvement associated with proliferative LN presents with nephritic syndrome and deterioration of renal function. The clinical and urinary finding usually correlates well with glomerular histological findings. Sometimes SLE may present with tubular dysfunction such as renal tubular acidosis. A renal biopsy is often useful to determine the histological class, whether the disease is active (potentially treatable) and choose treatment protocol or chronic and irreversibly scarred. Corticosteroids are a major component of treatment in the maintenance phase. Osteoporosis and AVN of bone are not uncommon in SLE patients. Women with SLE have five times higher fracture rates than normal women. Therefore, steroid dose should be minimized and vitamin-D and calcium supplements should be used to minimize bone loss.

FREQUENTLY ASKED QUESTIONS

Q1. How AVN of femoral head is diagnosed?

Ans. Initially, it may be asymptomatic. Subsequently, there may be mild-to-severe pain in the groin, thigh, or buttock. There may be limping gait. Appropriate imaging which includes X-ray, radionuclide bone scan, and MRI helps establishing the diagnosis.

Q2. What is the most sensitive test for AVN?

Ans. Magnetic resonance imaging of the hip joint is the most sensitive and specific test for diagnosis of AVN. The overall sensitivity is >90% and the specificity is also very high. The use of gadolinium is particularly useful in early detection.

Q3. What are the four stages of AVN?

Ans. Stage 1: Normal X-ray but MRI reveals the dead bone.

Stage 2: Can be seen on regular X-ray, but there is no collapse of the femoral head.

Stage 3: Shows signs of collapse (called a crescent sign) on X-ray.

Stage 4: Has collapse on X-ray and signs of cartilage damage (osteoarthritis).

Q4. What is the treatment of AVN?

Ans. In the early stages of AVN (precollapse), core decompression with or without bone graft. In advanced stage, total hip replacement may be done.

Membranous Nephropathy: Remission with Supportive Treatment

■ INTRODUCTION

Mr T, a 27-year-old nondiabetic, normotensive, nonsmoker, sand dredging laborer, was admitted with the complaints of generalized swelling for 4 months. He had been well until 4 months before this admission, when he developed swelling which appeared first on the face then became generalized. He also noted that his urine became frothy. Urine volume was normal.

He gave history of occasional low back pain which was noninflammatory in nature and usually occurred in the evening of his working days. He did not give any history of nonsteroidal anti-inflammatory drugs (NSAIDs) and as analgesic he only took acetaminophen. He had complaint of feverish feeling but fever was not documented. His appetite was good and bowel habit was normal. He had no history of skin rash, shortness of breath, burning sensation during urination, or passing dark urine.

He was diagnosed as a case of nephrotic syndrome (NS) having 24 hours urinary total protein (UTP) 10 g/day and bland sedimentation on urinalysis, with serum albumin 10 g/L and hypercholesterolemia. Secondary causes of glomerulonephritis were excluded based on absence of relevant positive clinical features and negative laboratory investigations. He then underwent renal biopsy. His serum creatinine was 1.5 mg/dL, normal C3, C4 level, negative antinuclear antibody (ANA), antids-DNA, perinuclear antineutrophil cytoplasmic antibody (p-ANCA), and cytoplasmic antineutrophil cytoplasmic antibodies (c-ANCA).

He was given ramipril and loop diuretics pending renal biopsy report.

Renal biopsy yielded 10 glomeruli, revealing:
- *Glomerulus*:
  - Size—enlarged
  - Cellularity—normocellular

- ○ Matrix—mildly increased (1+)
- ○ Glomerular basement membrane (GBM)—mildly thick
- *Tubules*:
  - ○ T atrophy
  - ○ *Epithelium*: Features of protein reabsorption
  - ○ *Tubular basement membrane (TBM)*: Normal
  - ○ *Cast*: Hyaline
- *Interstitium*:
  - ○ *Inflammation*: Mild, chronic
  - ○ *Fibrosis*: Mild
- *Blood vessels*: Unremarkable
- *Direct immunofluorescence (DIF)*:
  - ○ *Immunoglobulin G (IgG)*: Granular pattern—2+
- *Comment*: Compatible with membranous nephropathy (MN)

Correlating these biopsy findings with clinical presentation, a diagnosis of MN was made. Possible secondary causes were excluded. In order to substantiate the diagnosis of primary MN, phospholipase A2 receptor antibody titer was done which yielded negative result. With this massive proteinuria, immunosuppressives were being contemplated. But surprisingly, after 3 weeks of follow-up with antiproteinuric drug, his proteinuria decreased 5 g/day with normal renal function and improvement of serum albumin level to 35 g/L.

Although proteinuria was in the nephrotic range, owing to this excellent response to antiproteinuric, decision was taken to continue the patient on conservative management and follow-up closely. Dose of ramipril was increased.

His swelling subsided and general well-being also improved, except low back pain. After consultation with rheumatologist, the pain was attributed to his occupation and change of occupation was advised. He was not given any prophylaxis for thromboembolism.

■ DISCUSSION

All patients with primary MN and proteinuria should receive optimal supportive care. Immunosuppressive therapy is not required in patient with MN, NS, and normal estimated glomerular filtration rate (eGFR) unless atleast one-risk factor for disease progression or serious complications of NS. Many patients with primary MN and NS develop spontaneous remission. Data from randomized controlled trial (RCT) and cohort studies show favorable outcome (with spontaneous remission in up to 40%) in patients with MN and even at least one-risk factor with or without immunosuppressive therapy. If no risk factor is present and no complication of NS is evident, the use of immunosuppressive therapy rather adds some risk.

FREQUENTLY ASKED QUESTIONS

Q1. **When a kidney biopsy could be avoided in a suspected case of MN?**

Ans. Kidney biopsy is not required to confirm the diagnosis of MN in patients with NS and a positive antiphospholipase A2 receptor (PLA2R) antibody test.

Q2. **What are the sensitivity and specificity of positive antiPLA2R antibody test for diagnosis of primary MN?**

Ans. The sensitivity of a positive antiPLA2R antibody test for diagnosis of MN is 64% and specificity is 99%.

Q3. **What are the chances of spontaneous remission in MN?**

Ans. There is a 45% chance of spontaneous remission in patients with proteinuria >4 g/day after 6 months of conservative therapy, a 34% chance of spontaneous remission in patients with proteinuria >8 g/day for >6 months, 25–30% chance despite high urinary excretion of low molecular weight protein, and a 17% chance in patients in the upper tertiles of antiPLA2R antibody levels.

Collagenofibrotic Glomerulopathy

■ INTRODUCTION

Mrs NK, a 36-year-old homemaker, diagnosed as a case of hypothyroidism, hypertension, and chronic kidney disease (CKD) for 4 months, developed high-grade fever, vomiting, diarrhea, and decreased urine output 1 week following her second dose of COVID vaccination (with Moderna vaccine). Previously, she was on conservative treatment for her illnesses with serum creatinine around 3.2 mg/dL. However, renal function was not evaluated pre- and post-first dose vaccination or before second-dose vaccination. With these complaints, she was hospitalized and her serum creatinine was found to be 7.8 mg/dL **(Tables 1 and 2)**, which increased further and she needed two sessions of hemodialysis with two units blood transfusions. Renal function improved with conservative management in the following 2 weeks and she was discharged home with serum creatinine 3.7 mg/dL.

During routine follow-up 2 weeks later, she was found to have developed anorexia and vomiting and her serum creatinine was found to be 7.5 mg/dL along with proteinuria and she was readmitted. Considering the novel nature of the condition, after discussing with the patient and her attendants, decision was taken to treat her as a case of rapidly progressive glomerulonephritis. We treated her with intravenous (IV) methylprednisolone 1 g daily for 3 days followed by oral prednisolone 1 mg/kg/day. Serum creatinine decreased to 2.8 mg/dL in 1 week. We decided to continue oral steroid, added tablet telmisartan and discharged. Although she discontinued steroid by herself for a week, it was reinitiated during follow-up and continued. Tablet mycophenolate mofetil was also added to this regimen.

With this treatment, her serum creatinine came down to 1.64 mg/dL over the next 2 months. But, proteinuria persisted and she underwent renal biopsy.

Biopsy report shows:
- Glomerulopathy with marked mesangial expansion, nodular accentuation, and segments of capillary wall thickening
- Moderate interstitial scarring (30–40%)
- *Comment*: The histological features are suspicious for a deposition disease.

Electron microscopy:
- Up to four glomeruli were ultrastructurally examined, which showed mesangial expansion with presence of randomly arranged collagen fibers
- These long and thick fibers appeared focally curvilinear and in stacked bundle arrangements. Glomerular basement membrane (GBM) thickness appeared within normal limits. Podocytes showed segmental foot process effacement. Electron-dense immune complex type deposits were not seen. Tubules were not diagnostic.

Final diagnosis: Based on the histological and ultrastructural evaluation collagenofibrotic/type III collagen glomerulopathy is a likely diagnosis.

Medication list:
- Tablet prednisolone—30 mg at morning (after meal)
- Tablet levothyroxine sodium—50 µg at morning 1 hour before breakfast
- Tablet prazosin 2.5 mg XR—twice daily
- Tablet nifedipine SR 20 mg—thrice daily
- Tablet bisoprolol 5 mg—twice daily
- Tablet telmisartan 80 mg—once daily
- Tablet calcium acetate 667 mg—twice daily with food
- Injection erythropoietin 5,000 IU—subcutaneous (SC) every 7 days
- Capsule carbonyl iron + folic acid + zinc—once daily
- Tablet febuxostat 40 mg—once daily
- Tablet rabeprazole 20 mg—once daily before meal
- Tablet domperidone 10 mg—thrice daily before meal
- Tablet cholecalciferol 1,000 IU—once daily.

Investigation Profile (Tables 1 and 2)

TABLE 1: Urinalysis and renal function test.	
Protein	++
RBC (/HPF)	6–10
WBC (/HPF)	20–25
Cast (/LPF)	Nil
UTP (g/day)	5.06
UTV (mL/day)	2,500

Continued

Continued

Urine C/S	No growth
S. Creatinine (mg/dL)	7.8
Na$^+$ (mmol/L)	141
K$^+$ (mmol/L)	5.3
Cl$^-$ (mmol/L)	98
T-CO$_2$ (mmol/L)	21

(HPF: high power field; LPF: low power field; RBC: red blood cell; UTP: urinary total protein; UTV: urinary total volume per day; WBC: white blood cell)

TABLE 2: Other laboratory investigations.	
Hb	7.4 g/dL
ESR	133 mm in 1st hour
TC	6,000/µL
N/L/M/E (%)	80/14/04/02
Platelet	160,000/µL
PBF	Combined deficiency anemia
Serum iron	8.2 µg/dL
TIBC	15 µg/dL
Serum ferritin	1,723 ng/mL
TSAT	54%
Calcium	7.03 mg/dL
Phosphate	5.4 mg/dL
Uric acid	5.57 mg/dL
iPTH	
Albumin	3.5 g/dL
SGPT	19 U/L
RBS	7.2 mmol/L
TSH	2.91 ulU/mL
FT4	1.07 ng/dL
ANA	Negative
Anti-ds-DNA	Negative
C3	Low
C4	Normal
p-ANCA	Negative

Continued

Continued

c-ANCA	Negative
HBsAg	Negative
Anti-HBC	Negative
Total cholesterol	192 mg/dL
HDL cholesterol	47 mg/dL
LDL Cholesterol	138 mg/dL
Triglycerides	172 mg/dL

(ANA: antinuclear antibody; C-ANCA: cytoplasmic antineutrophil cytoplasmic antibody; ESR: erythrocyte sedimentation rate; Hb: hemoglobin; HBC: hepatitis B core antigen; HDL: high-density lipoprotein; iPTH: intact parathyroid hormone; LDL: low-density lipoprotein; P-ANCA: perinuclear anti-neutrophil cytoplasmic antibody; PBF: peripheral blood film; RBS: random blood sugar; SGPT: serum glutamic pyruvic transaminase; TC: total count; TIBC: total iron-binding capacity; TSH: thyroid-stimulating hormone)

Ultrasonography of Kidney, Ureter, and Bladder Region

- *Impression*: Bilateral renal parenchymal change

DISCUSSION

Collagenofibrotic glomerulopathy (CFG) is a rare condition caused by mesangial and subendothelial deposition of collagen type III in glomeruli. Collagen type III is not a normal constituent of the extracellular matrix of glomeruli, but it is found in the interstitium and vessel wall. Clinical features of CFG include proteinuria (often in nephrotic range) edema and hypertension. The condition can progress to end-stage kidney disease, requiring dialysis, or renal transplantation.

Mesangial cell could be responsible for the accumulation of collagen III caused by glomerular injury and/or cytokine stimulation, Human complement factor H deficiency, hemolysis, and hemolytic uremic syndrome are also associated with the causation of CFG. In our case, it is unclear whether COVID vaccine caused glomerular injury and/or cytokine stimulation causing deposition of type III collagen in the subendothelial space and mesangium. With regard to COVID vaccination, the preclinical trials have shown that MRNA vaccine caused strong CD4+ and CD8+ T cell response, antibody response, and cytokine release.

As reported by most recent literature, both messenger RNA (MRNA) and inactivated vaccine could be involved in causation of nephropathy either after the first or second dose. Reported nephropathies were minimal change disease (MCD), immunoglobulin A nephropathy (IgAN), membranous nephropathy (MN), focal segmental glomerulosclerosis (FSGS), and systemic vasculitis. Immunoglobulin A (IgA) nephritis showed a rapidly progressive course consistent with the presence of crescents on renal biopsy. Some patients presented with severe renal failure due to tubulointerstitial nephritis (TIN) after COVID vaccination. With regard to prognosis, some patients with TIN and severe renal failure require hemodialysis and had complete recovery of renal function under glucocorticoid treatment. Patients with rapidly progressive IgAN and severe renal failure improved after hemodialysis; however, it is not possible to conclusively determine whether there is a causal relationship between severe acute respiratory syndrome coronavirus 2 (SARS CoV-2) vaccination and new-onset nephropathies based on urinary abnormalities and/or renal insufficiency shortly after vaccination. One can presume that immune response to the COVID-19 vaccine may be a trigger of nephropathies.

FREQUENTLY ASKED QUESTIONS

Q1. What is collagenofibrotic glomerulopathy?

Ans. It is a rare cause of idiopathic nephrotic syndrome characterized by massive accumulation of atypical type III collagen fibrils within mesangial matrix and subendothelial space of the glomeruli.

Q2. What are the glomerular diseases associated with vaccination?

Ans. MCD, IgAN, IgAN with crescent [rapidly progressive glomerulonephritis (RPGN)], anti-GBM nephritis, MN, and FSGS. Systemic vasculitis has been found to occur after COVID vaccination. Acute TIN has also been reported.

Q3. What are the patterns of onset of glomerulonephritis after SARS CoV-2 vaccination?

Ans. Glomerulonephritis may be of new onset or relapsing type after COVID-19 vaccination.

Cytomegalovirus Pneumonia in Kidney Transplant Patient

◼ INTRODUCTION

Mr AH, a 46-year-old man, underwent renal transplantation with the background diagnosis of glomerulonephritis (GN), hypertension (HTN), and end-stage renal disease (ESRD) on hemodialysis (HD). Donor was his younger sister. There were three antigen mismatches. Donor and recipient were both cytomegalovirus (CMV) immunoglobulin G (IgG) positive. The perioperative period was uneventful, except for persistently raised blood glucose. Warm ischemic time was 45 seconds and cold ischemic time was 30 minutes. His immunosuppressive regimen comprised of induction with two doses of basiliximab, injectable methylprednisolone followed by oral prednisolone, cyclosporine, and mycophenolic acid (MPA). He was discharged 4 weeks after the transplant with a serum creatinine (S. Cr) of 1.5 mg/dL.

A week after discharge, he presented with abdominal discomfort and hiccup. Abdominal examination was normal and blood pressure was 140/90 mm Hg. There were no signs of steroid or cyclosporine toxicity. S. Cr was 1.6 mg/dL, which rose to 2.5 mg/dL in the next week. By that time, he also developed cough and respiratory distress with a persistently low oxygen saturation of 80–85%, which was clinically diagnosed as acute respiratory distress syndrome (ARDS) based on X-ray **(Fig. 1)** and computed tomography (CT) chest findings **(Fig. 2)**. Total count of white blood cell (WBC) was 3,800/cumm, erythrocyte sedimentation rate (ESR) was 10 mm in the 1st hour, and serum electrolyte was normal. No evidence of infection was found on urine routine examination (RE), urine and blood culture, dengue NS1 antigen, and sputum for acid-fast bacillus (AFB) and GeneXpert. CMV IgM and CMV DNA were found to be positive.

Therefore, injectable ganciclovir was started with a diagnosis of CMV pneumonia and isolation was maintained as much as possible. Mycophenolate acid (MPA) was put on hold, but other immunosuppressive

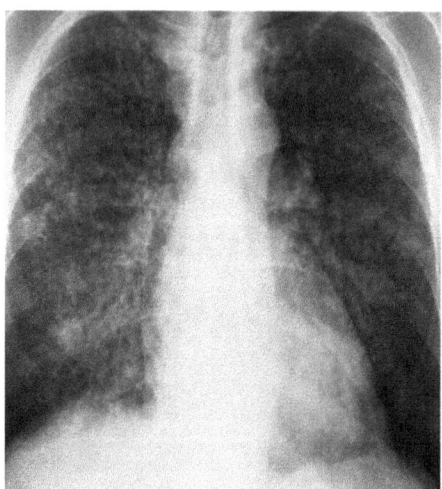

FIG. 1: Chest X-ray posteroanterior (PA) view—bilateral reticulo-interstitial infiltrations, especially in right mid and lower zone.

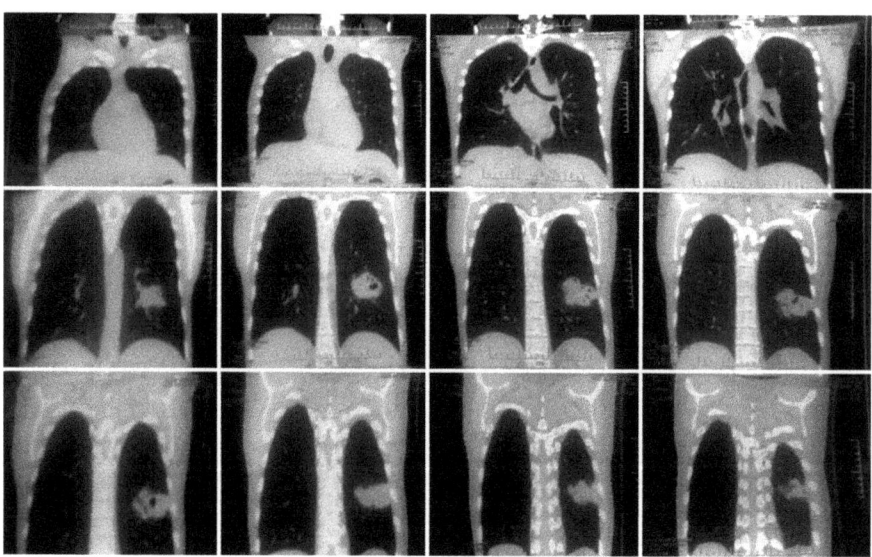

FIG. 2: Computed tomography (CT) scan of the chest—extensive patchy regions of ground glass density in both lungs.

drugs were continued. After continuing ganciclovir for 67 days, CMV DNA became undetectable, when ganciclovir was stopped. His serum creatinine gradually came down to normal over the course of this treatment and he was clinically improved.

■ DISCUSSION

Cytomegalovirus infection is a frequent complication after transplantation, especially up to 100 days post-transplant. Infection usually occurs due to transmission from transplanted organ, due to reactivation of latent infection, or after a primary infection in a seronegative patient. Therefore, factors that influence CMV infection are the CMV serostatus of recipient and donor, use of lymphocyte depleting agents, level of immunosuppression, and donor type (living or deceased). CMV infection is defined as isolation or detection of viral proteins (antigens) or nucleic acid in any body fluid or tissue specimen regardless of symptoms or signs. CMV disease may be defined as presence of appropriate clinical symptoms and/or signs together with documentation of CMV in tissue from the relevant organ by histopathology, virus isolation, rapid culture, immunohistochemistry, or DNA hybridization unless there are data supporting that other materials can be accepted as having similar significance. It is recognized that high viral DNA levels detected with quantitative nucleic acid test (NAT), polymerase chain reaction (PCR) in tissue from relevant organ likely represent CMV disease. For example, in a case of CMV pneumonia (as is our case), symptoms and/or signs of pneumonia such as new infiltrates on imaging, hypoxia, tachypnea, and/or dyspnea combined with CMV documented in lung tissue by virus isolation, rapid culture, histopathology, immunohistochemistry, or DNA hybridization technique.

During symptomatic CMV infection, kidney transplant (KT) recipients may experience fever, leukopenia, diarrhea, hepatitis, colitis, or allograft injury. These KT recipients have an increased susceptibility to opportunistic infections, increased risk of acute rejection, diminished graft survival, higher incidence of chronic allograft nephropathy, and decreased patient survival rate. Currently, treatment of CMV infection varies from center to center; however, two strategies are acceptable. According to guideline, universal prophylaxis and preemptive therapy. Universal prophylaxis involves the administration of antiviral medication to all patients or subset of at-risk patients. Antivirals are usually started in the immediate post-transplant period and continued for 3–6 months. For preemptive therapy, the patients are monitored regularly for CMV infection and treatment is started once active viral replication is evident. Preemptive protocol utilizes a variety of tests for detection of CMV PP 65 antigen, DNA, or mRNA to diagnose and monitor therapeutic response to CMV infection. Under this protocol, treatment is continued until two consecutive negative antigenemia assay results obtained. Patient with CMV infection should receive intravenous ganciclovir or oral valganciclovir for a minimum of 14 days until resolution of symptoms.

FREQUENTLY ASKED QUESTIONS

Q1.   What is the mortality rate of CMV infection in transplant patient?

Ans. The mortality of primary CMV infection is about 54% and associated with a significantly higher rate of pulmonary super infection in the first year after transplantation.

Q2.   How common is CMV infection in transplant patients?

Ans. Between 20 and 60% of people with a solid organ transplant develop a symptomatic CMV infection.

Q3.   Why CMV infection occurs in KT?

Ans. Cytomegalovirus is a globally widespread virus that becomes latent following primary infection but reactivates frequently and causes disease in KT recipients in the setting of immunosuppression.

Cellular Rejection in Renal Allograft Recipient

▌ INTRODUCTION

M J, 33-year-old, renal allograft recipient for last 3 years, hypertensive, nondiabetic, presented with the complaints of generalized weakness for 15 days. According to the statement of the patient, he was reasonably well 15 days back. Then he developed generalized weakness which was mild and associated with malaise and lassitude. With this complaint and as a part of routine evaluation for transplant kidney, he was investigated and found to have significant renal impairment with a serum creatinine of 7.2 mg/dL, which rose to 9.5 mg/dL over a period of weeks. He got admitted in a tertiary care hospital and was treated with injection methylprednisolone 500 g daily for 5 days followed by oral prednisolone 20 mg daily and his serum creatinine came down to 6.3 mg/dL. He was then transferred to the university hospital for further evaluation and management. His weakness was not preceded by any fever, cough, diarrhea, vomiting, or use of nephrotoxic medication. He does not give any history of passage of dark color urine, reduction of volume of urine (average urine output was 1,200–1,500 mL/day), dysuria, loin pain, or generalized swelling. There is no history of skin rash, oral ulcer, photosensitivity, arthralgia, or abdominal pain.

In 2018, he was diagnosed as a case of glomerulonephritis (based on proteinuria and hematuria), hypertension, and chronic kidney disease (CKD). Serum creatinine was 3 mg/dL at presentation. He was treated conservatively and did not undergo renal biopsy. Over a period of 1 year, his serum creatinine rose to 13 mg/dL and he underwent renal transplantation **(Tables 1 to 4)** with three to four sessions of hemodialysis before transplantation. There is no history of blood transfusion. He cannot mention his induction therapy, but maintenance was given with mycophenolate mofetil (MMF), tacrolimus, and steroid. His serum creatinine came down to 1.3 mg/dL within a week of transplant. Prophylaxis with valganciclovir and cotrimoxazole was given.

He was on tacrolimus 6 mg daily, MMF 1,000 mg daily, and tablet prednisolone 5 mg daily. He was on regular follow-up, although he admits taking immunosuppressive drugs irregularly on few occasions, at times stop them for up to 3–4 days due to difficulty in obtaining drugs. Despite that, his post-transplant period was uneventful. Serum creatinine always remained near baseline. There were no episodes suggestive of acute rejection or any infectious complications that needed treatment. There is no similar sort of illness running in the family.

He is a nonsmoker and nonalcoholic. He belongs to middle class family and is immunized according to Expanded Programme on Immunization (EPI) schedule. He has not received any adult vaccination, except hepatitis B vaccine (HBV) vaccine.

■ EXAMINATION

General Examination

- Conscious, oriented, and co-operative
- Anemia +
- Nonicteric
- *Weight*: 55 kg
- *Pulse*: 76 beats/min, regular
- *Blood pressure (BP)*: 120/80 mm Hg
- *Temperature*: 98.2° F
- *Respiratory rate*: 18 breaths/min
- No lymphadenopathy
- *Thyroid gland*: Not enlarged
- *Jugular venous pressure (JVP)*: Not raised
- *Edema*: Absent
- *Skin condition*: Normal
- Bedside urine dipstick reveals +++ proteinuria

Abdominal Examination

- *Inspection*: Normal in shape
- *Palpation*: Soft, nontender, no graft tenderness, and no organomegaly
- *Percussion*: No evidence of ascites
- *Auscultation*: Bowel sound present

Respiratory System

- *Inspection*: Normal
- *Palpation*: Trachea central in position.
  - Apex beat palpable at left 5th inhaled corticosteroids (ICS) medial to midclavicular line

- *Percussion*: Resonant
- *Auscultation*: Breath sound vesicular

Other systems including fundoscopy reveal no abnormalities.

Ongoing Medications

- Tab tacrolimus 1 mg 3 + 0 + 3
- Tab MMF 500 mg 1 + 0 + 1
- Tab prednisolone 20 mg 1 + 0 + 0
- Tab prazosin XR 2.5 mg 1 + 0 + 1
- Tab amlodipine 5 mg 0 + 0 + 1
- Tab bisoprolol 5 mg 0 + 0 + 1
- Tab sodium bicarbonate 600 mg 1 + 0 + 1

DIAGNOSIS

Renal allograft recipient, hypertension, and for the current presentation, differentials are:
- Recurrent glomerulonephritis with crescentic transformation
- De novo glomerulonephritis
- Transplant glomerulopathy
- Acute rejection

INVESTIGATIONS

TABLE 1: Recipient and donor workup.		
	Recipient	**Donor**
Blood group	O positive	O positive
CMV IgG	Reactive	Reactive
CMV IgM	Negative	Negative
Cross matching	Negative	Negative
HLA 1 and 11 antibody	Negative	
DSA class 1 DSA class 11	Negative	
Rejection or infective episodes	No	
Induction ATG	Given	

(ATG: antithymocyte globulin; CMV: cytomegalovirus; DSA: donor-specific antibodies; IgG: immunoglobulin G; IgM: immunoglobulin M; HLA: human leukocyte antigen)

TABLE 2: Urine test.	
Protein	++
RBC	Nil
WBC	1–2/HPF
Cast	Nil
UTP	4.12 g/24 hours
UTV	2,500 mL
Urine C/S	No growth

(HPF: high power field; RBC: red blood cell; UTP: urinary total protein; UTV: urinary total volume; WBC: white blood cell)

TABLE 3: Renal function test and complete blood count (CBC).	
S. creatinine (mg/dL)	9.09 (injection methylprednisolone 1 g daily started)
S. urea (mg/dL)	97
S. Na	140
S. K	3.5
S. Cl	103
S. TCO_2	24.67
Hb (g/dL)	12.60 g/dL
ESR (mm in 1st hour)	42
WBC/cumm N/L/M/E%	7,970 74/18/05/03
Platelet (cumm)	207,000

(ESR: erythrocyte sedimentation rate; Hb: hemoglobin; WBC: white blood cell; S.: serum)

TABLE 4: Other laboratory parameters.	
P-ANCA	2.85 (negative)
C-ANCA	3.12 (negative)
ANA	Negative
C3 (80–170 mg/dL)	0.859 g/L
C4 (20–50 mg/dL)	0.522 g/L
CRP	<3.12 mg/L
Serum ferritin	553.5 ng/mL on
BT	2 minutes 30 seconds
CT	5 minutes 45 seconds
PT	10.60 seconds
APTT	27 seconds
HBsAg	Negative

Continued

Continued

Anti-HCV	Negative
Anti-CMV IgG	118 IU (positive)
Anti-CMV IgM	Negative
RBS	9.4 mmol/L
HbA1c	6.2%
Serum albumin	36 g/L
LDH	277 U/L
Vitamin D level	34.08 ng/mL
Bilirubin	0.4 mg/dL
ALT	12 U/L
Serum phosphate	7.1 mg/dL
Serum calcium	1.8 mmol/L
Serum uric acid	7 mg/dL
Tacrolimus trough level	5.7 ng/mL 4.8 ng/mL
PCR for CMV	Pending
PCR for BK virus	Pending

(ALT: alanine transaminase; ANA: antinuclear antibody; APTT: activated partial thromboplastin time; BT: bleeding time; C-ANCA: cytoplasmic antineutrophil cytoplasmic antibody; CMV: cytomegalovirus; CRP: C-reactive protein; CT: clotting time; HCV: hepatitis C virus; LDL: low-density lipoprotein; P-ANCA: perinuclear antineutrophil cytoplasmic antibody; PCR: polymerase chain reaction; PT: prothrombin time; RBS: random blood sugar)

Doppler Ultrasonography of Transplant Kidney (Figs. 1A and B)

Clinical history: Transplanted kidney.

Findings

B-mode Imaging

Transplanted kidney measurements about 9.0 cm. Cortical thickness (16 mm) is within normal limits. Cortical echogenicity is mildly increased. Cortex and medulla are well-defined. Pelvicalyceal system is not dilated. No perinephric collection is noted.

Doppler Imaging

RI of interlobar artery is 0.70.
PSV in renal artery at anastomotic site is 48 cm/s with evidence of turbulence. Renal vein have color flow and phasicity. No thrombus is detected in renal vein.

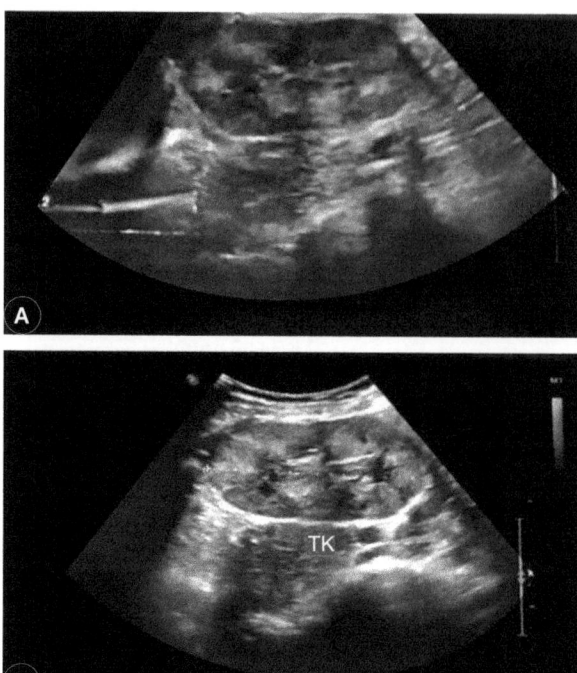

FIGS. 1A AND B: Ultrasonography (USG) of transplant kidney.

Color Doppler of Transplant Kidney

Kidney size >> almost normal in size, shows normal parenchymal thickness but echogenic parenchyma and mildly impaired cortical medullary differentiation.

No calculus or calyceal dilatation or any focal mass seen in it. The perinephric spaces are clear. No evidence of fluid collection seen.

(Size of kidney 10.7 × 5.5 cm, parenchyma: 1.8 cm, location right iliac area).

Ureter: Not dilated

On color Doppler:
- Normal arterial pulsations seen at renal hilum
- Blood flow study was performed from the site of anastomosis of renal artery, infundibular vessels up to arcuate arteries.
- Shows normal vascular flow and wave pattern with normal peak systolic velocity (PSV)'s but mildly increased resistive index (RI) in all arteries on spectral Doppler (RI of IIA—0.9, LA—0.63, ILA—0.79, ARC art—0.62).

Comment:
>> Echogenic parenchyma and mildly impaired cortical medullary differentiation seen in transplanted kidney and mildly increased RI seen in all the arteries >> *Suggest of chronic parenchymal insufficiency*

Impression

Renal and intrarenal arterial flow are within normal limits.

◼ TRANSPLANTED KIDNEY BIOPSY REPORT

Gross Examination

Specimen consists of linear core of tissue measuring 0.7 × 0.2 cm.

Microscopic Appearance

Section shows renal tissue containing 16 glomeruli and four arterial sections. One of the glomeruli is globally sclerosed. The other shows mild increase in mesangial cells and matrix. The glomerular basement membrane is focally thick with double contours in about 10% of glomeruli. Mild glomerulitis is present in some of the glomeruli. Mild peritubular capillaritis is seen in <10% of the cortex. Interstitial fibrosis with tubular atrophy and mild inflammation is seen involving >25% of cortical interstitium, mild tubulitis is seen in the fibrosed areas. Arteries show mild thick wall with intimal fibrosis with about 5% narrowing of the lumen. No endothelialitis is seen. Few arterioles with noncircumferential hyaline are seen.

Dx: Suggestive of cellular rejection, grade 1A.

◼ DISCUSSION

Rejection, acute, or chronic is diagnosed by histologic finding after transplant kidney biopsy. A biopsy considered adequate where the sample contains at least 10 glomeruli and two small arteries. A biopsy specimen with seven to nine glomeruli and one artery is considered marginal. When biopsy is performed for clinical indications, two separate cores should be obtained. Another name for cellular rejection is T-cell-mediated rejection. The classification of T-cell-mediated rejection (cellular rejection) is based on the degree and location of mononuclear cell inflammation. The predominant phenotypes of cell are CD4+ and CD8+ T-cells, B-cells, eosinophils, and monocytes may also be present. When interstitial inflammation is severe, it involves the tubules [tuberculous meningitis (TBM)] causing tubulitis (when lymphocytes and monocytes extend into the walls and lumen of tubules), the histologic finding of endothelialitis (T-cells and macrophages extend under arterial endothelium) is pathognomonic of acute cellular rejection. Typically, C4D staining is negative. In acute cellular rejection, endothelialitis may or may not be accompanied by interstitial inflammation or tubulitis. Acute T-cell-mediated rejection is classified on the basis of presence or absence of endothelialitis, the degree of interstitial inflammation, and quantity of infiltrating cells in tubules. For example, type I acute cellular rejection is characterized by absence of endothelialitis, with interstitial inflammation of at least 25% of the parenchyma, tubulitis, and in type II and type III acute cellular rejection, vascular involvement (endothelialitis) is a characteristic feature. Chronic active T-cell-mediated rejection is characterized by arterial intimal fibrosis with evidence of mononuclear cell infiltration and formation of neo intima. The primary diagnostic assessment includes history especially adherence to immunosuppressive protocol, physical examination, blood and urine laboratory tests, measurement of serum level of drugs, and ultrasonography.

Diagnosis of acute cellular rejection depends on biopsy, CD20 staining for refractory cases, negative C4D staining, presence of markers of activated lymphocytes, and proteomic study. Treatment of acute cellular rejection in kidney transplant recipient includes pulse steroid for first rejection. For recurrent or resistant rejection, thymoglobulin and OKT3 are used as the second line of treatment; if graft function is deteriorating. Changing the protocol from cyclosporine to tacrolimus or adding mycophenolate mofetil or sirolimus might be effective. Prognosis depends on number of rejection episodes, the use of potent drugs, the time of rejection from transplantation, and response to treatment.

FREQUENTLY ASKED QUESTIONS

Q1. What are signs and symptoms of acute rejection?

Ans. Fever, flu-like symptoms, chills, aches, headache, nausea, and/or vomiting decreased urine output, swelling of body, new pain, or tenderness around the transplant kidney.

Q2. How is acute cellular rejection treated?

Ans. Intravenous methylprednisolone 500 mg daily for 3–5 days. ATG or OKT3 may also be used.

Q3. How can you prevent acute rejection?

Ans. The use of a brief course of potent immunosuppression at the time of transplantation, referred to as induction therapy, has become a common strategy for the prevention of acute rejection.

Vascular Complication after Renal Transplantation

◼ INTRODUCTION

Mr MA, 28-year-old male with a primary diagnosis of glomerulonephritis, hypertension, and chronic kidney disease, on maintenance hemodialysis for 2 years underwent live related renal transplantation. Patient had very high blood pressure, which was difficult to control with highest doses of oral nifedipine, prazosin, bisoprolol, and losartan along with clonidine as needed. Preoperative urine output was almost nil. Iliac and femoral vessels were normal on duplex study.

Donor was his maternal cousin, Mr AR, 28-year-old male. Both donor and recipient were blood group O positive. There were three antigen mismatches, one each in A, B, and DR **(Table 1)** and negative B and T cell cross match. Both donor and recipient were cytomegalovirus (CMV) immunoglobulin G (IgG) positive. There were no cardiac or other relevant issues in donor or recipient. There were single renal arteries and veins. ^{99m}Tc-diethylenetriaminepentaacetate (DTPA) renogram was normal.

TABLE 1: Human leukocyte antigen (HLA) typing.		
HLA typing	**Donor**	**Recipient**
A	A11, A3	A11, A33(19)
B	B52(5), B–	B52(5), B44(12)
DR	DR10, DR7	DR10, DR15(2)

Cytotoxic (T-cell and B-cell) cross match:
- *T-cell cross match*: Negative
- *B-cell cross match*: Negative

The intraoperative period was uneventful from the surgical side. The warm ischemic time was 30 seconds and cold ischemic time was 86 minutes (including a perfusion time of 22 minutes). Injection methylprednisolone and basiliximab induction was given in the intraoperative period. From anesthesiologic side, blood pressure was persistently high around 200–220/100–120 mm Hg during the surgery and recipient needed intravenous (IV) antihypertensives. Reversal was uneventful. Maintenance immunosuppressives consisted of oral steroid, tacrolimus, and myco-phenolate mofetil.

In the immediate postoperative period, his urine output was 300 mL in the first 4 hours, but it fell to below 5 mL/hour in the subsequent period. There was severe pain in the graft site, which persisted for 36 hours following surgery and subsided little with opioid. Blood pressure remained high and patient needed IV antihypertensives in the form of glyceryl trinitrate (GTN) and labetalol. Serum creatinine rose from 6.25 mg/dL preoperative to 10.6 mg/dL on the second postoperative day (POD) **(Table 2)**. Hemodialysis was started. Hemoglobin fell from 9.5 preoperative to 7.6 in 2 days **(Tables 3 and 4)**. Two units of red cell concentrates (RCC) were given using leukocyte filter after excluding autoimmune hemolysis.

Anuria persisted. There was no fever or signs of systemic upset. Urinary catheter obstruction was excluded. Ureteric obstruction by possible urinoma or lymphocele was also excluded via ultrasound. Ultrasound using power Doppler on the first POD showed no arterial flow in the interlobar and arcuate arteries and minimal arterial flow in the segmental artery, where resistivity index was 1.0. There was <50% stenosis at the arterial

TABLE 2: Graft function.		
	Before KT	**After KT**
S. creatinine (mg/dL)	6.25	10.6
Na$^+$ (mmol/L)	138	130.4
K$^+$ (mmol/L)	4	4.8
Cl$^+$ (mmol/L)	98	96.6
TCO$_2$ (mmol/L)	22	23

TABLE 3: Complete blood count (CBC).	
Hb (g/dL)	7.4
ESR (mm in 1st hour)	08
TC	8,300
DC (%) (N/L/M/E)	94/05/01/00
Platelet (/mm^3)	170,000

(ESR: erythrocyte sedimentation rate; DC: differential count; Hb: hemoglobin)

anastomotic site with turbulent flow. Renal vein showed no evidence of thrombus. A similar picture persisted on repeat ultrasound on the 3rd and 9th POD. Computed tomography (CT) renal angiography was done on 5th POD, which showed <50% narrowing at the arterial anastomotic site, but no kinking. There was opacification of the segmental and interlobar arteries, but no excretion of contrast media, second dose of basiliximab was given on 4th POD and rest of the immunosuppressives were continued for a month. But there was no sign of graft function and the patient remained dialysis-dependent. Decision was taken to stop mycophenolate mofetil, decrease the dose of tacrolimus, and continue along with low-dose steroid considering the possibility of retransplantation.

TABLE 4: Other laboratory parameters.	
Blood C/S	No growth
Serum bilirubin (T)	0.3 mg/dL
Serum bilirubin (D)	0.18 mg/dL
ALT (SGPT)	60 U/L
LDH	794 U/L
Reticulocyte count	3.56×10^9/L
hsCRP	99.82 mg/L
Procalcitonin	8.7 µg/L
D-dimer	3.2 µg/mL
RBS	5.6 mmol/L
Fibrinogen	424 mg/L (200–400)
PT	12.6 seconds (12–16)
APTT	32 seconds (20–40)
Coombs test (direct and indirect)	Negative
Calcium	10.8 mg/dL
Albumin	42 g/L
Phosphate	12.4 mg/dL
Serum iPTH	2,280 pg/mL
Vitamin-D level	
Serum iron	6.2 µmol/L
TIBC	36 µmol/L
TSAT	17.2%
Serum ferritin	471 ng/mL

(ALT: alanine transaminase; APTT: activated partial thromboplastin time; hsCRP: high-sensitivity C-reactive protein; LDH: lactate dehydrogenase; iPTH: intact parathyroid hormone; PT: prothrombin time; RBS: random blood sugar; SGPT: serum glutamic pyruvic transaminase; TIBC: total iron-binding capacity; TSAT: transferrin saturation)

Doppler Ultrasonography on 1st Postoperative Day

Clinical history: Transplanted kidney

Findings
- *B-mode imaging*: Transplanted kidney measurements about 10.0 cm. Cortical thickness (15.2 mm) is within normal limits. Cortical echogenicity is normal. Cortex and medulla are well-defined. Pelvicalyceal system is not dilated. No perinephric collection is noted.
- *Doppler imaging*: No arterial flow observed in interlobar and arcuate arteries even in power Doppler. Minimal arterial flow seen in segmental artery.
- Resistive index (RI) of segmental artery is 1.00.
- Peak systolic velocity in renal artery at anastomotic site is 30 cm/s with evidence of turbulence.
- Renal vein have color flow and phasicity.
- No thrombus is detected in renal vein.

Impression
- No arterial flow observed in interlobar and arcuate arteries even in power Doppler. Minimal arterial flow in segmental artery.
- <50% stenosis at anastomotic site of renal artery

Doppler Ultrasonography on 3rd Postoperative Day

Clinical history: Transplanted kidney

Findings
- *B-mode imaging*: Transplanted kidney measurements about 9.3 cm. Cortical thickness (12.4 mm) is within normal limits. Cortical echogenicity is normal. Cortex and medulla are well-defined. Pelvicalyceal system is not dilated. No perinephric collection is noted.
- *Doppler imaging*: No arterial flow observed in segmental, interlobar, and arcuate arteries even in power Doppler.
- Peak systolic velocity in renal artery at anastomotic site is 113 cm/s with evidence of turbulence.
- Renal vein have color flow and phasicity. No thrombus is detected in renal vein.

Impression
- No arterial flow observed in intrarenal arteries even in power Doppler
- 50–70% stenosis at anastomotic site of renal artery

Doppler Ultrasonography on 9th Postoperative Day

Clinical history: Transplanted kidney

Findings
- *B-mode imaging*: Transplanted kidney measurements about 9.4 cm. Cortical thickness (12.5 mm) is within normal limits. Cortical echogenicity is mildly increased. Cortex and medulla are well-defined with prominent pyramids.
- Pelvicalyceal system is not dilated. No perinephric collection is noted.

- *Doppler imaging*: RI of interlobar artery is 1.0.
- Peak systolic velocity in renal artery at anastomotic site is 49.7 cm/s with evidence of turbulence.
- Renal vein have color flow and phasicity. No thrombus is detected in renal vein.

Impression
- Increased resistance in intrarenal arteries
- <50% stenosis at anastomotic site of renal artery

Computed Tomography Renal Angiogram on 5th Postoperative Day

Multiple axial noncontrast and contrast CT scan were performed.

Findings

Renal artery of transplant kidney anastomosis with right external iliac artery. Mild narrowing (<50%) is seen at anastomotic site. However, no evidence of kinking is noted. Segmental and interlobar arteries are well-opacified but no appreciable excreting of the contrast media is noted. No significant abnormality is detected in renal and internal iliac vein.

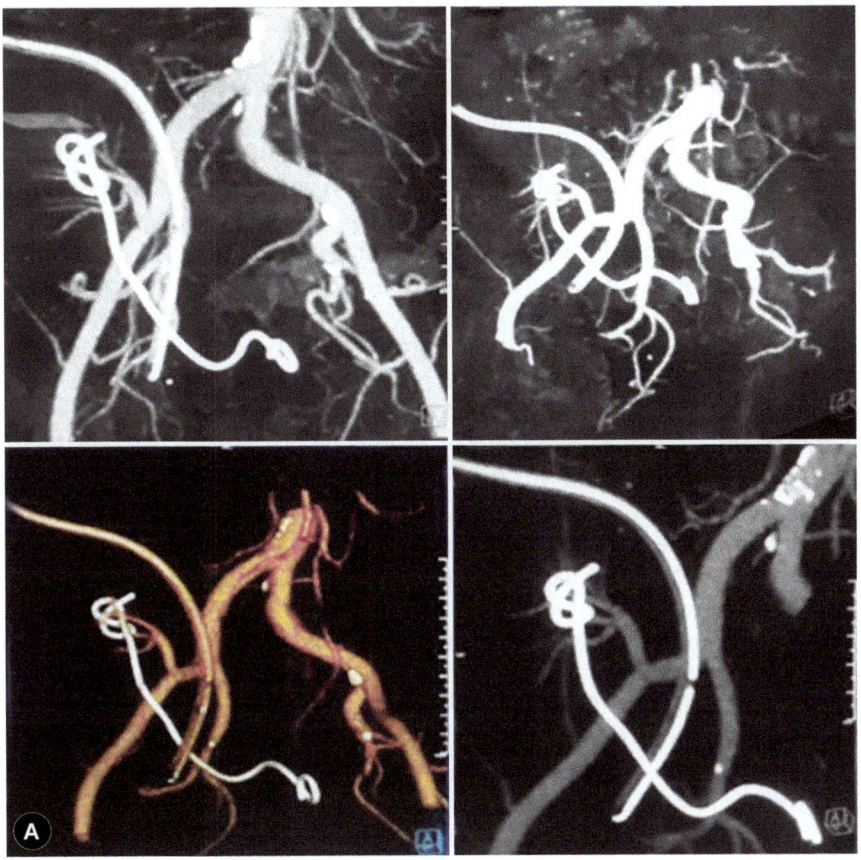

Continued

Continued

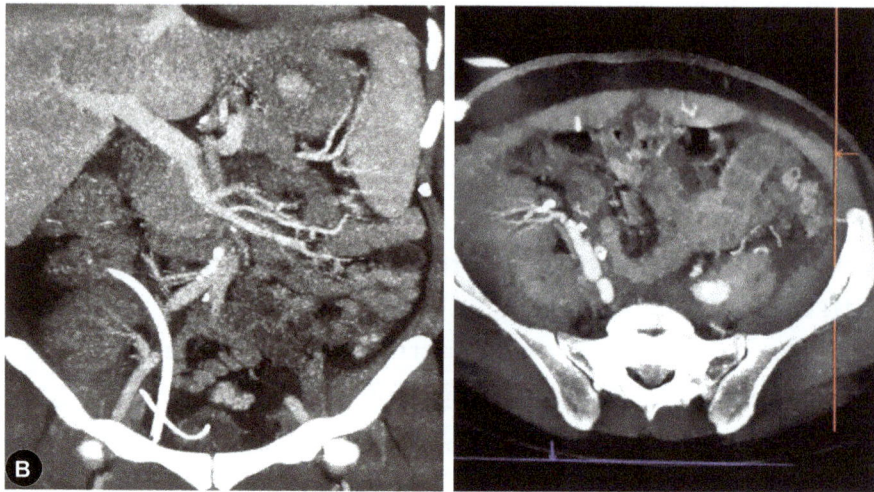

FIGS. 1A AND B: Computed tomography (CT) renal angiogram of transplant kidney.

■ DISCUSSION

In the early era of kidney transplant, surgical complications were a major cause of graft loss. Between 1960 and 1980, the estimated incidence was around 20%. With the improvements of surgical techniques, the frequency of these complications has dropped significantly. Currently, the incidence of surgical complications is <5%. In general, the results of renal transplantation have improved primarily as a consequence of advances in medical and immunosuppressive therapy and progress in surgical techniques. In most of the series post-transplant, urological complications are in the range of 2.5 to 27% and causes significant morbidity and mortality. Surgical complications after renal transplantation can be classified mainly as vascular (arterial and venous thrombosis renal arterial stenosis, lymphocele, and hemorrhage) and urologic (ureteral obstruction, vesicoureteric reflux, and urinary fistula). Theoretically, there is a greater risk of surgical complications associated with living donors and recipients of kidneys with multiple arteries. Therefore, there is a need for close attention to the anatomy of the donor due to possibility of having two or more arteries and veins, or early arterial bifurcation. The most worrisome of vascular complication is arterial thrombosis (about 1%); during nephrectomy and perfusion, injury may occur in the endothelial layer facilitating the process of thrombosis. The anastomoses of small vessels of different sizes or twisting or bending pressure are other predisposing factors for thrombosis. The hallmark of renal artery thrombosis is the absence of blood perfusion of the parenchyma which can still be identified intraoperative. In the postoperative period, the most common clinical presentation is the sudden interruption of urine flow without pain in the graft.

The renal perfusion should be evaluated by dimercaptosuccinic acid (DMSA) renal scintigraphy, by ultrasound Doppler and even with arteriography. Immediate surgical exploration may be done in few cases, especially if the diagnosis of arterial thrombosis is done before closing the incision. The loss of the graft is the most common consequence and nephrectomy should be performed.

FREQUENTLY ASKED QUESTIONS

Q1. What are the common vascular complications after renal transplantation?

Ans. Common vascular complications are transplant renal artery stenosis, transplant renal artery thrombosis, transplant renal vein thrombosis, biopsy-induced vascular injury, pseudoaneurysm formation, and hematoma.

Q2. What is the most common vascular complication following renal transplant?

Ans. Transplant renal artery stenosis is the most common vascular complication. It occurs in 3–23% in first 12 months.

Q3. What is the prognosis of transplant renal vein thrombosis?

Ans. Transplant renal vein thrombosis usually occurs early after surgery in 0.1–4.2% cases. Diagnosis depends on high index of suspicion and a quick duplex study. Very early thrombolytic therapy or surgical thrombectomy may be tried, but the usual end result is graft loss.

Sepsis in a Renal Allograft Recipient

■ INTRODUCTION

Patient Md RAL, 49-year-old overseas worker, hypertensive for 16 years, diabetic for 3 years, a live related renal transplant recipient 10 years back, on a background diagnosis of autosomal dominant polycystic kidney disease (ADPKD), hypertension, chronic kidney disease (CKD) presented to us with the complaints of gradual deterioration of renal function for 5 months.

He was diagnosed as a case of ADPKD 17 years back, although none of his family members were found to have a similar condition. There was no history suggesting neurological complications. Since then he was on conservative management. Six years later, his renal function started deteriorating. Renal transplantation was done the next year.

Donor was his younger sister. There were three antigen mismatches. Both donor and recipient had blood group match and were cytomegalovirus (CMV) immunoglobulin G (IgG) positive. He cannot mention his induction therapy, but maintenance was done with mycophenolate mofetil (MMF), tacrolimus, and prednisolone. His discharge creatinine was 1.5 mg/dL. He was compliant with his treatment and was on regular follow-up. Serum creatinine was maintained close to discharge creatinine. Five years later, MMF was switched to azathioprine to curtail expenses. But 1 year later, he developed severe anemia and needed blood transfusion, at which point azathioprine was switched back to MMF. There were no episodes or hospitalizations suggestive of acute rejection.

For the last 5 months, he has been experiencing gradual deterioration of renal function. Serum creatinine rose from a baseline of 1.8 to 5.6 mg/dL over 4 months. Upon evaluation, tacrolimus trough level was found to be low, which came back to normal after dose adjustment. But after admission, he developed pain and swelling in his right leg along with high-grade remittent fever. Highest recorded temperature was 102°F. Peripheral pulsation was intact. He also developed shortness of breath and needed oxygen supplement to maintain saturation.

He is hypertensive for 15 years and on nifedipine, bisoprolol, and prazosin. He was found to be diabetic on his routine follow-up 3 years back. He was initially put on oral antidiabetic drugs but later switched to insulin. There were no hypoglycemic or hyperglycemic emergencies and no macro- and microvascular complication except nonproliferative diabetic retinopathy. He was recently diagnosed as a case of hypothyroidism and on supplement.

On examination, he was anemic, blood pressure (BP) 130/80 mm Hg with medication, SpO_2 98% with 2 L/min O_2, bedside urine dipstick test reveals +++ proteinuria. There was swelling, redness, and tenderness and raised temperature present over-the-outer side of the right leg. Two blackish areas were present **(Fig. 1)**.

Investigation revealed hemoglobin (Hb) 7.2 g/dL, erythrocyte sedimentation rate (ESR) 29, white blood cell (WBC) count 3,800, platelet count 80,000, C-reactive protein (CRP) 66.6 mg/L, serum ferritin 1,539 ng/mL, urine R/E—protein ++, pus cell 6–10/high power field (HPF), red blood cell (RBC) nil, urinary total protein (UTP) 4.4 g/24 hours.

Considering cellulitis, injection meropenem 500 mg intravenous (IV) 12 hourly and injection amoxicillin and clavulanic acid 0.6 g IV 12 hourly were started empirically. With no improvement over the next 4 days, injection vancomycin 1 g stat and 500 mg IV every 3rd day was prescribed in place of injection amoxicillin and clavulanic acid. Surgical consultation was taken and deep vein thrombosis (DVT) was excluded via duplex ultrasonography.

Despite all efforts, his condition deteriorated rapidly. A diagnosis of sepsis was made and hemodialysis (HD) was initiated. Following the second HD session, he suddenly lost consciousness. On evaluation, he was found to have planter extensor bilaterally, jerks increased, pin point pupil, and rapidly falling oxygen saturation. Urgent intensive care unit (ICU) referral

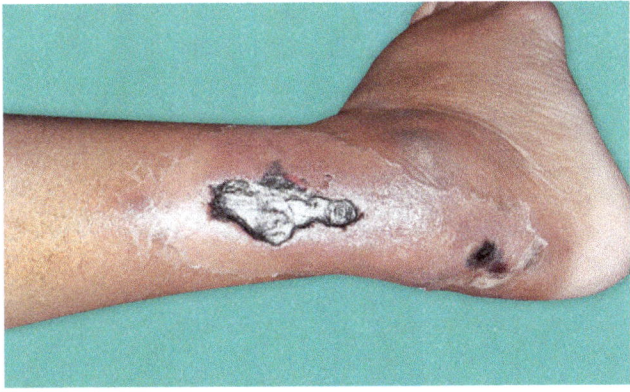

FIG. 1: Swelling, redness, and blackish area on leg.

was given. But the patient expired before any further interventions could be arranged.

DISCUSSION

Infection is the most common noncardiac cause of death after solid organ transplant, and sepsis is a major hurdle to disease-free survival after renal transplantation. About 70% of renal transplant recipients have at least one episode of infection within 3 years of receiving the transplant.

Hospital mortality in renal transplant patients with severe sepsis and septic shock is associated with male gender, worst SOFA score on admission and presence of hematologic dysfunction, mechanical ventilation, and advanced graft dysfunction.

FREQUENTLY ASKED QUESTIONS

Q1. What is the leading cause of death in renal transplant patients?

Ans. Infection has been the major cause of death in renal transplant patients.

Q2. Can organs be donated during sepsis?

Ans. Bacteremia or bacterial sepsis precludes organ donation.

Q3. What are the common causes of infection in transplant recipient in the immediate postoperative period?

Ans. Bacterial infection including vascular, other nosocomial infection (including pneumonia), *Clostridium difficile* colitis, and surgical site infection.

Chronic Pyelonephritis due to Vesicoureteric Reflux, Secondary FSGS, Renal Abscess, and CKD

■ INTRODUCTION

Mrs HA, 24-year-old homemaker was admitted with the complaints of fever and dysuria for 7 days and generalized swelling for 3 years. Fever was high grade, remittent in nature associated with occasional chills and rigors and a highest recorded temperature of 102°F. Dysuria was associated with frequency, urgency, flank pain, and vomiting.

She gives history of similar episodes of urinary tract infection (UTI) for the last 8 years, occurring about two to four times per year, occasionally culture proven. Each time she was treated with intravenous (IV) or oral antibiotics and the symptoms improved. Three years back, she developed bilateral renal abscess and had to undergo Double-J (DJ) stenting temporarily. At that time during further evaluation, she was diagnosed as a case of vesicoureteric reflux (VUR) based on history of repeated UTIs, ultrasonography, uroflowmetry **(Fig. 1)**, and micturating cystourethrogram. Ureteroneocystostomy was done on the left and planned for the right, but she did not comply. She did not experience any UTI-like episode in the subsequent 3 years.

About two and half years ago, she developed generalized swelling and upon evaluation was found to have nephrotic syndrome. Urinary total protein was 3.6 g/day and serum creatinine rose from 1.8 to 3.8 mg/dL. Renal biopsy was advised, but she refused. She was put on conservative management, but renal function progressively deteriorated.

She has two children. There is no family history of similar illness.

On examination, she is mildly anemic and bedside urine reveals ++ protein.

She is currently on IV ceftriaxone for UTI along with antihypertensives and conservative management for chronic kidney disease (CKD).

■ INVESTIGATIONS (TABLES 1 TO 3 AND FIG. 1)

TABLE 1: Urine R/E, urine C/S, blood C/S, complete blood count (CBC) and renal function test.	
Pus cell	20–30/HPF
Epithelial cells	10–15/HPF
RBC	2–5/HPF
Protein	++
Sugar	Nil
Sp gravity	1.010
Urine (C/S)	*Escherichia coli* >10^5
Blood (C/S)	No growth
Hb	10.4 g%
ESR	36 mm in 1st hour
TC	9×10^9
N	73%
L	26%
MCV	87.3 fl
MCH	28.2 pg
RDW-CV	13.2%
Urea	56 mg/dL
Creatinine	6.7 mg/dL

(ESR: erythrocyte sedimentation rate; HRF: high power field; MCH: mean corpuscular hemoglobin; MCV: mean corpuscular volume; RBC: red blood cell; RDW-CV: coefficient of variation red cell distribution width)

TABLE 2: Others laboratory parameters.	
Serum Na$^+$	138 mmol/L
Serum K$^+$	3.9 mmol/L
Serum Cl$^-$	103 mmol/L
T-CO$_2$	14 mmol/L
Serum vitamin D	22 ng/mL
Serum uric acid	7.10 mg/dL
Serum albumin	37 g/L
Serum PTH	132.7 pg/mL
Serum inorganic phosphate	6.5 mg/dL
Serum calcium	8.0 mg/dL
Serum magnesium	2.20 mg/dL
eGFR	8 mL/min/1.73 m^2

(eGFR: estimated glomerular filtration rate; PTH: parathyroid hormone)

TABLE 3: Other serological tests.	
CRP	10.9 mg/L
ANA	Negative
HLA B27	Negative
Anti-SM	Negative
Anti-SSA	Negative
Anti-SSB	Negative

(CRP: C-reactive protein; HLA: human leukocyte antigen)

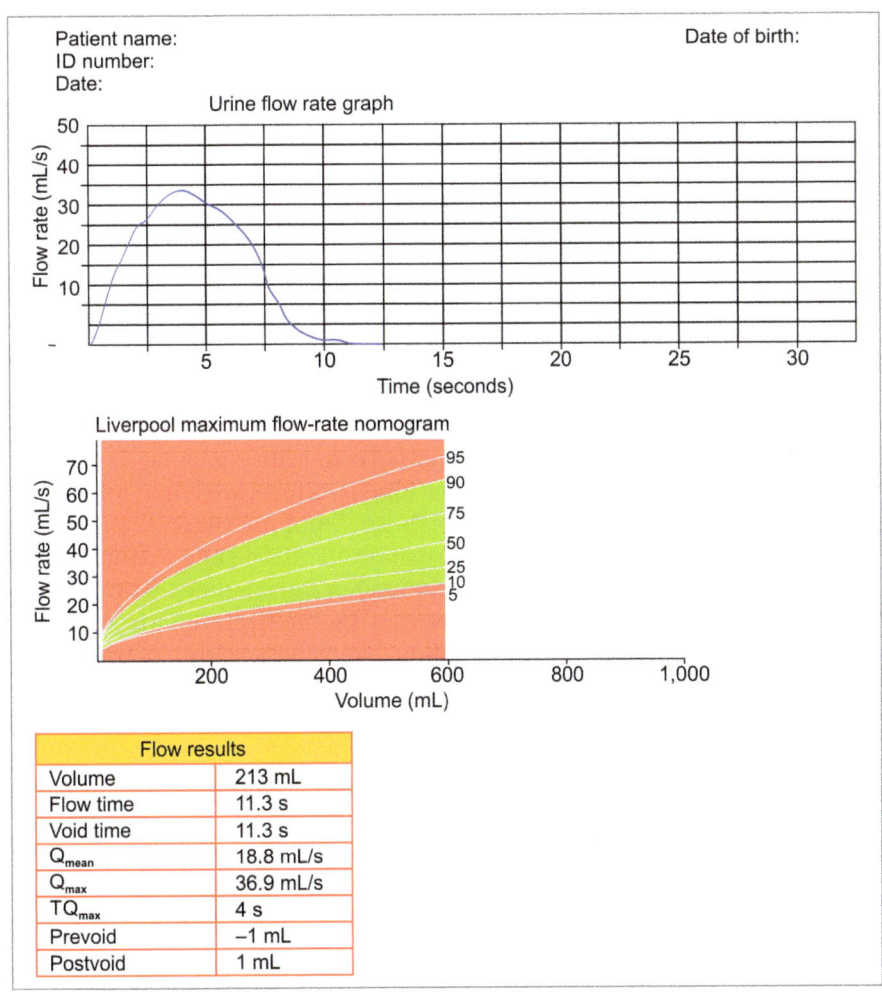

FIG. 1: Uroflowmetry.

Ultrasonography of Kidney, Ureter, and Bladder Region

Bipolar diameter of right kidney 9 cm, left kidney 9.3 cm, pelvicalyceal system dilated on left side.

Ureter: Dilated on left side.

Parenchyma: Cortical echogenicity increased, corticomedullary differentiation reduced. Isoehoic areas detected on both side.

Impression: Bilateral parenchymal disease. Bilateral renal abscess.
- *Urine GeneXpert for MTB*: Not detected
- Micturating Cysto-Urethrogram (MCU)
  - Chronic bladder outlet obstruction
  - B/L VUR
    - Hypertrophy of bladder neck; cystitis
    - B/L VUR-grade IV at right and grade V at left

X-ray both sacroiliac (SI) joints anteroposterior (AP) and Ferguson view: Bilateral sacralization
- Computed tomography (CT) scan of whole abdomen
  - B/L small kidneys with left-sided hydronephrosis
  - Thick-walled urinary bladder—cystitis

A clinical diagnosis of chronic pyelonephritis, VUR, secondary focal segmental glomerulosclerosis (FSGS), renal abscess, and CKD was made.

▌DISCUSSION

Vesicoureteric reflux is a condition where there is retrograde flow of urine from bladder to kidneys. It may be congenital or hereditary. It may be primary (an isolated abnormality) or secondary (due to other congenital anomalies of the kidney and urinary tract such as renal dysplasia, obstructive uropathy-neurogenic bladder). VUR is usually identified by fetal ultrasound (dilatation of fetal renal pelvis in pregnancy) or during diagnostic work-up of UTI in children. Due to VUR, there may be recurrent UTI in children. Recurrent infection and intrarenal reflux can cause scarring of the kidney (reflux nephropathy).

The presentation of reflux nephropathy may be in the form of recurrent UTI, hypertension, chronic pyelonephritis, CKD, etc. Intrarenal reflux causes parenchymal injury and patients may present with proteinuria due to secondary FSGS.

Management includes treatment of UTI and long-term chemoprophylaxis until resolution of VUR. Surgical treatment is recommended in case of high-grade VUR having attacks of UTI in spite of chemoprophylaxis and in case of noncompliance with medical management.

FREQUENTLY ASKED QUESTIONS

Q1. Classify VUR.

Ans.

Grade	Degree of VUR
I	Ureter only
II	Reflux into ureter, pelvis, and calyces with no dilatation and normal calyceal fornices
III	Mild or moderate dilatation of ureter, pelvis, and calyces with no or slight blunting of fornices
IV	Moderate dilatation and tortuosity of ureter, moderate dilation of pelvis and calyces. Complete obliteration of sharp angles of fornices, but maintenance of papillary impression
V	Gross dilatation and tortuosity of ureter, pelvis, and calyces. Papillary impression no longer visible

Q2. How long it takes renal scarring to occur?

Ans. It may take several years (may be about 6 years) from discovery of VUR to appearance of renal scar.

Q3. Is infection is always required for renal scarring to occur?

Ans. In some, renal scarring may occur without infection, especially in male with severe VUR-associated renal dysplasia. These are usually boys with primary congenital grade IV or V VUR. Most commonly in female children, a combination of recurrent upper UTI and VUR causes renal scarring.

Refractory Lupus Nephritis

▍INTRODUCTION

Mr ST, a 20-year-old normotensive, nondiabetic student, presented with the complaints of generalized swelling for 7 days along with high color scanty micturition for same duration. He noticed swelling around the eyes and face and progressively became generalized by 7 days. However, swelling was not preceded by fever, sore throat or any skin infection. He complains of passage of dark color urine for the same duration which is not associated with burning sensation during micturition or loin pain. There is no history of chest pain, shortness of breath, cough, jaundice, oral ulcer, photosensitivity, abdominal pain, arthralgia, or bloody diarrhea. There was no family history of similar type of illness.

Two years back, he was evaluated for skin lesion involving oral cavity and ear and was diagnosed as systemic lupus erythematosus (SLE) with lupus nephritis (LN) having proteinuria with active urine sediments **(Table 1)**. He did not undergo renal biopsy and there is no medical record of that time. One year later, he was found to have renal impairment associated with other laboratory findings **(Tables 2 and 3)** during follow-up. Later on he underwent renal biopsy which revealed class 4 LN **(Table 4)** and was treated with intravenous (IV) methylprednisolone for 3 days followed by oral prednisolone along with injectable cyclophosphamide pulse fortnightly. His renal function was not improving despite this treatment, he developed shortness of breath and abnormal behavior. At that point, he received three sessions of plasma exchange and intravenous immunoglobulin (IVIg) along with three sessions of hemodialysis. His symptoms subsided and renal function became normal. Since his medical records are not available, the possible indications of plasmapheresis and IVIg were thought to be alveolar hemorrhage and severe neuropsychiatric manifestations.

He was put on mycophenolate mofetil (MMF) along with steroid as maintenance therapy. He was in complete remission for 1 year. Four months back, he again developed rapid deterioration of renal function. There was preceding history of potentially acute kidney injury (AKI) precipitating events. He was then admitted to a tertiary care center. Hemodialysis was started along with IV methylprednisolone for 3 days followed by oral prednisolone and fortnightly pulse injectable cyclophosphamide. His renal function was declining and he was admitted to our center. After detailed evaluation and discussion with the patient, three sessions of plasma exchanges were given considering a possible refractory LN. His serum creatinine came down to 2.2 mg/dL. He was discharged with fortnightly pulse cyclophosphamide and oral steroid.

EXAMINATION

General Physical Examination
- Conscious, oriented, and cooperative
- Anemia—absent
- Nonicteric
- Weight—95 kg
- Pulse—70 bpm, regular
- Blood pressure (BP)—140/90 mm Hg
- Temp—98.2°F
- Respiratory rate—18 breaths/min
- No lymphadenopathy
- Thyroid gland—not enlarged
- Jugular venous pressure (JVP)—not raised
- Edema—bilateral pitting pedal edema present
- Bedside urine dipstick reveals +++ *proteinuria*

Examination of others system revealed no abnormalities.

Provisional Diagnosis
Systemic lupus erythematosus with LN with flare.

Investigations

TABLE 1: Urinalysis.	
Protein	+++
RBC	Plenty
Pus	15–20/HPF
Cast	Nil
UTP	5.99 g/day
UTV	800 mL/day

(HPF: high power field; RBC: red blood cell; UTP: urinary total protein; UTV: urinary total volume)

TABLE 2: Complete blood count (CBC).			
Hemoglobin (Hb)	11.3 g/dL		
ESR	10 mm in 1st hour		
WBC	14,000/cmm	N	92%
		L	06%
		E	00%
		M	02%
		B	00%
Platelet	2,20,000/cmm		

(WBC: white blood cell; ESR: erythrocyte sedimentation rate)

TABLE 3: Renal function test and other biochemical parameters.	
Serum creatinine	7.35 mg/dL
Serum sodium (Na^+)	140 mmol/L
Serum potassium (K^+)	5.25 mmol/L
Serum chloride (Cl^-)	107 mmol/L
Serum TCO_2	26 mmol/L
Serum Ca	1.9 mmol/L
Serum PO_4	5.8 mmol/L
RBS	5.4 mmol/L
Serum C3 (80–170 mg/dL)	30 mg/dL
Serum C4 (20–50 mg/dL)	7 mg/dL
Serum albumin (38–50 g/L)	23 g/L

TABLE 4: Renal biopsy report.			
Light microscopic examination (Received in 10% formalin)			
Glomerulus	Number	8	*Crescent*: Cellular (1/8)
	Size	Enlarged	
	Cellularity	Proliferation of endocapillary and mesangial cells	
	Matrix	Increased	
	GBM	Mildly thick	
	Additional findings	Inflammatory cells with nuclear debris	
Tubule	Epithelium	Features of protein reabsorption	*Tubulitis*: Present *Others*: Focal tubular injury
	Cast	RBC, hyaline	
Inflammation	Chronic inflammatory cells including eosinophils		Edema
Blood vessels	Thick walled	Mildly thick	*Vasculitis*: Mild features of vasculitis

Continued

Continued

DIF funding (Received in normal saline)					
Deposited antibody	IgG	IgM	IgA	C3	C1q
Site of deposition	Capillary wall and mesangium	Capillary wall and mesangium	Capillary wall and mesangium	Capillary wall and mesangium	Capillary wall and mesangium
Pattern of deposition	Granular	Granular	Granular	Granular	Granular
Intensity	4+	4+	4+	4+	4+

(DIF: direct immunofluorescence; GBM: glomerular basement membrane; IgA: immunoglobulin A; IgG: immunoglobulin G; IgM: immunoglobulin M; RBC: red blood cell)

◾ DISCUSSION

Refractory LN indicates an inadequate response to treatment. That means persisting or worsening disease activity despite treatment. Understanding the causes of refractory disease and developing treatment strategies is important because these patients are more likely to develop poor outcome, especially end-stage kidney disease.

Treatment options include higher doses of glucocorticoid, switching between cyclophosphamide and mycophenolic acid derivative or addition of rituximab, belimumab, or voclosporin. Other options may be plasma exchange or immunoadsorption, calcineurin inhibitors, and IVIg.

FREQUENTLY ASKED QUESTIONS

Q1. What is the best medication for LN?

Ans. Treatment options include glucocorticoids, cyclophosphamide, azathioprine, mycophenolic acid derivative, calcineurin inhibitors, rituximab, etc. Belimumab and voclosporin are Food and Drug Administration (FDA) approved, specifically for refractory LN.

Q2. What is refractory LN?

Ans. Refractory LN, broadly defined as failure to attain clinical remission after appropriate induction immunosuppressive therapy, is associated with an increased risk of progression to end-stage kidney disease and mortality. Refractory disease is generally assessed on the basis of clinical parameters, which may be unreliable and renal biopsy, which is not often performed in a standard or timely fashion. So, there is a lack of international consensus regarding what constitutes a refractory disease.

Q3. What is SLEDAI score ?

Ans. Disease activity in LN has been defined on the basis of SLEDAI scores: No activity (SLEDAI = O), mild activity (SLEDAI = 1–5), moderate activity (SLEDAI = 6–10), high activity (SLEDAI = 11–19), and very high activity (SLEDAI ≥20).

Systemic Amyloidosis Involving Kidney and Heart

■ INTRODUCTION

Mrs MB, 40-year-old normotensive, nondiabetic homemaker, presented to us with the complaints of generalized swelling and scanty micturition for 5 months and left-sided weakness for 3 days. Swelling was occasionally associated with frothy urine.

She also complained of occasional dyspnea, orthopnea, and paroxysmal nocturnal dyspnea, which has been increasing in severity for the last few weeks. Now she experiences breathlessness even on mild exertion. This is associated with occasional palpitation. Three days ago, she developed sudden weakness of left side of the body along with facial deviation to the right while getting up from bed in the morning. It was not associated with vomiting, convulsion, or loss of consciousness.

She does not give any history of joint pain, skin rash, oral ulcer, cold intolerance, intake of any nephrotoxic or herbal medications, blood transfusion, and history of renal disease in her family. However, she has two siblings who died at the age of 43 and 46 years from cardiac events. She is amenorrheic for the last 8 months.

On general examination, she has hyperpigmentation present on her forehead, redness of right eye, and bilateral pedal edema. Bedside urine revealed ++ proteinuria. Other parameters of general examination including jugular venous pressure (JVP) are within normal limits.

On nervous system examination, speech is slurred, but higher cerebral function is intact with a Glasgow Coma Scale (GCS) score of 15. Fundoscopy is normal. There is upper motor type of facial nerve palsy on the left side and extensor planter response on the left. Respiratory system examination reveals bilateral pleural effusion. Other systemic examinations including cardiovascular system examination reveal normal findings.

Investigations reveal bland urine with urinary total protein (UTP) of 2.6 g/day [urinary total volume (UTV): 900 mL], with a corresponding serum albumin of 1.3 g/dL. Serum creatinine gradually rose from 0.65 to 1.64 mg/dL over the course of this illness. Ultrasonography revealed normal sized kidneys with increased cortical echogenicity and poor corticomedullary differentiation. Chest X-ray revealed bilateral pleural effusion. Echocardiogram showed global hypokinesia [left ventricular ejection fraction (LVEF): 34%], concentric left ventricular hypertrophy (LVH), mild mitral regurgitation (MR), tricuspid regurgitation (TR), and diastolic dysfunction in restrictive pattern. It was suggestive of amyloidosis.

Markers for secondary causes of glomerulonephritis, along with multiple myeloma, were excluded. Renal biopsy was performed, which showed:

- *Light microscopy*:
  - Glomeruli
  - Size—enlarged
  - Cellularity—not increased
  - Matrix—increased (+3)
  - Glomerular basement membrane (GBM)—mild irregularly thick
  - Sclerosis—4/8 global, 2/8 segmental
  - Crescents—none
  - Tubules
  - Tubular atrophy—mild
  - Epithelium—features of protein reabsorption
  - Cast—hyaline, granular
  - Interstitium
  - Inflammation—moderate, chronic
  - Fibrosis—moderate
  - Blood vessels
  - Thick-walled
  - Hyaline arteriosclerosis
  - Congo red stain: Amyloid deposition in the mesangium and blood vessels

DIRECT IMMUNOFLUORESCENCE

Only 3+ deposit of lambda in smudgy pattern in mesangium and blood vessels. Consultation was taken from Department of Hematology and decision was taken to shift the patient for further management. But the patient decided to discontinue treatment and discharged herself against medical advice.

DISCUSSION

Amyloidosis is a rare disease that occurs when amyloid proteins are deposited in tissues and organs. Amyloid proteins are abnormal proteins, which the body cannot breakdown. When amyloid proteins clump together, they form amyloid deposits. Amyloidosis most frequently affects the kidneys, heart, nervous system, liver, and gastrointestinal tract. The buildup of these amyloid deposits damage organs and tissues.

When deposited in kidneys, it causes proteinuria and/or hypertension followed by progressive renal failure. Four types of amyloidosis most often affect the kidneys:

1. Immunoglobulin light-chain amyloidosis (AL amyloidosis) or primary amyloidosis
2. AA amyloidosis or secondary amyloidosis—often associated with certain chronic inflammatory conditions
3. Leukocyte cell-derived chemotaxin 2 (LECT 2); most commonly affects kidneys and liver
4. Hereditary amyloidosis, due to rare gene mutations

▌ TREATMENT

High-dose chemotherapy with stem cell transplant is the treatment of choice.

Treatment of Primary Amyloidosis (AL Amyloidosis)

The four drug combination of subcutaneous daratumumab, bortezomib, cyclophosphamide, and dexamethasone is safe and effective. United States (US) Food and Drug Administration approved tafamidis meglumine (Vyndaqel) and tafamidis (Vyndamax) for cardiomyopathy caused by transthyretin-mediated amyloidosis (ATTR CM).

FREQUENTLY ASKED QUESTIONS

Q1. What is the treatment of systemic amyloidosis?

Ans. High-dose chemotherapy followed by autologous bone marrow transplantation.

Q2. What is the treatment of dialysis related amyloidosis?

Ans. Renal transplant

Q3. What are the complications of renal amyloidosis?

Ans. Renal scarring, anemia, bone disease, hypertension, and chronic kidney disease (CKD).

Myelodysplastic Syndrome and Nephrotic Syndrome

■ INTRODUCTION

Md MR, 60-year-old farmer, hypertensive for 4 years, nondiabetic, presented with the complaints of generalized swelling along with frothy urine for 2 months. Swelling was not preceded by fever, sore throat, skin infection or associated with burning sensation during micturition, or loin pain. There is no history of dyspnea, orthopnea, paroxysmal nocturnal dyspnea, jaundice, cough, hemoptysis, altered bowel habit, or weight loss. He was found to have nephrotic range proteinuria and was admitted for renal biopsy. After admission upon further evaluation **(Tables 1 and 2)**, he found to have anemia, leukocytosis, and thrombocytosis and splenomegaly. Based upon hematology consultation, examination of bone marrow aspiration and trephine biopsy was done and he was diagnosed as a case of myelodysplastic syndrome (MDS). There is no similar sort of illness running in the family. He gives no history of taking herbal or any nephrotoxic medications.

On examination, he is anemic, edematous, with a blood pressure (BP) of 140/90 mm Hg, but no lymphadenopathy. Bedside urine dipstick reveals +++ proteinuria. Systemic examination including fundoscopy reveals normal findings.

■ INVESTIGATIONS

TABLE 1: Urinalysis.	
Protein	++
Pus cell	0–2/HPF
RBC	Nil
Cast	Absent
Sugar	Nil
Urine C/S	No growth
Urinary total protein	6.8 g/day

(HPF: high power field; RBC: red blood cell)

TABLE 2: Complete blood count (CBC) and other laboratory parameters.			
Hemoglobin (Hb)	9.1 g/dL		
ESR	15 mm in 1st hour		
WBC	16,000/cmm	N	74%
		L	21%
		E	03%
		M	02%
		B	00%
Platelet	1,225,000/cmm		
Serum creatinine	2.21 mg/dL		
Serum sodium (Na$^+$)	144 mmol/L		
Serum potassium (K$^+$)	4.3 mmol/L		
Serum chloride (Cl$^-$)	108 mmol/L		
Serum TCO$_2$	23.2 mmol/L		
p-ANCA	Negative		
c-ANCA	Negative		
ANA	Negative		
C3 (80–170 mg/dL)	67 mg/dL		
C4 (20–50 mg/dL)	14 mg/dL		
Serum albumin (38–50 g/L)	37 g/L		
BT	2 minutes 15 seconds		
CT	5 minutes 10 seconds		
PT	15.60 seconds		

(ANA: antinuclear antibody; BT: bleeding time; c-ANCA: cytoplasmic antineutrophil cytoplasmic antibody; CT: clotting time; ESR: erythrocyte sedimentation rate; p-ANCA: perinuclear antineutrophil cytoplasmic antibody; PT: prothrombin time; WBC: white blood cell)

The patient was advised renal biopsy, but he denied. Several case reports are available regarding association between MDS and nephrotic syndrome. Most common histological variety was found to be membranous nephropathy and immunoglobulin A (IgA) nephropathy.

PROVISIONAL DIAGNOSIS

Glomerulonephritis (GN) (nephrotic presentation), hypertension (HTN), and MDS.

Ultrasonography of Whole Abdomen

- Liver is normal in size, parenchyma appears coarse in echotexture.
- Spleen is enlarged in size (14.3 cm) and uniform echopattern.

- Right kidney 9.5 cm, left kidney 9.6 cm, cortical echogenicity is increased, and corticomedullary differentiation (CMD) is poor.
- Prostate is enlarged in size with uniform echopattern, volume is about 38.8 cc.

BONE MARROW EXAMINATION REPORT

- *Site*: Posterior superior iliac spine
- *Consistency of bone*: Normal
- *Aspiration*: Easy
- *Cellularity*: Normocellular
- *M/E ratio*: Increased
- *Erythropoiesis*: Active and dimorphic
- *Granulopoiesis*: Active and maturing into segment form
- *Megakaryocytes*: Variable size with feature dysplasia seen
- *Lymphocytes*: Seen
- *Plasma cell*: Seen
- *Other cell lines*: Unremarkable
- *Comments*: Trilineage hematopoiesis dysplasia with trilineage dysplasia

HISTOPATHOLOGY REPORT

Specimen: Bone Tissue (Trephine Biopsy)

- *Gross examination*: Specimen consists of a linear gray white piece of tissue measuring 0.8 cm. Submitted as such after short decalcification.
- *Microscopic examination*: Sections show a core of spongy bone. The marrow cellularity is increased. Blast cells are slightly increased. Granulopoiesis is increased and erythropoiesis is active. Megakaryocytes are frequently seen and hypolobulated, some are atypical.

DISCUSSION

Kidney along with other organs is a target of autoimmunity in the setting of MDS. MDS is associated of several autoimmune kidney manifestation predominantly acute tubulointerstitial nephritis (TIN) and more rarely various immune GN. These may be membranous nephropathy, antineutrophil cytoplasmic antibody (ANCA)-negative pauci immune necrotizing and crescentic GN, C3 glomerulopathy, fibrillary GN, and immunoglobulin-associated membranoproliferative GN, which have been linked to autoimmune process.

Fibrillary GN probably results from glomerular deposition of immune complexes that have ability to undergo fibrillogenesis. However, the exact mechanisms underlying autoimmune manifestations in MDS patient remain speculative.

The treatment of nephropathies associated with MDS relies mostly on immunosuppressive treatments, which carry specific morbidity (mostly infections) and mortality. The use of cytotoxic drugs may lead to a worsening of MDS-associated cytopenias, rapid tapering of steroids, and, when feasible, the use of noncytotoxic agents (such as rituximab) is recommended in these patient. Our patient was treated with hydroxyurea.

FREQUENTLY ASKED QUESTIONS

Q1. How common is renal involvement in MDS?

Ans. Renal involvement in patients with MDS is rare; with a frequency from 0.48 to 4%.

Q2. What are the complications of MDS?

Ans.

- Anemia
- Recurrent infections
- Bleeding
- Increased risk of cancer

Q3. What are the patterns of renal involvement in MDS?

Ans. The patterns of renal involvement in MDS are:

- Acute TIN
- ANCA-negative pauci immune necrotizing and crescentic GN
- Membranous nephropathy
- IgA nephropathy
- Immunoglobulin-associated membranoproliferative GN
- Crescentic C3 glomerulopathy
- Fibrillary GN
- Minimal change disease

Q4. What is atheroembolic renal disease?

Ans. It usually occurs in older patients suffering from atherosclerosis and is a result of embolization of cholesterol crystals from atheromatous plaques in small-sized arteries. Acute renal failure of variable severity may occur. A common laboratory finding is eosinophilia, which may be an expression of MDS and GN may be a rare association.

Minimal Change Disease or Focal Segmental Glomerulosclerosis

■ INTRODUCTION

Ms R, 19-year-old, hypertensive, nondiabetic student, presented with a history of generalized swelling for 1 year. She was diagnosed as a case of glomerulonephritis 3 years back based on clinical presentation, proteinuria, and active urine sediment. Her urinary total protein (UTP) was 12 g/day and serum complements C3 and C4 were normal.

Secondary causes of glomerulonephritis were excluded based on absence of relevant clinical features and negative laboratory investigations [antinuclear antibody (ANA), anti-ds-DNA, anti-Sm, cytoplasmic anti-neutrophil cytoplasmic antibody (c-ANCA), perinuclear anti-neutrophil cytoplasmic antibody (p-ANCA), hepatitis B surface antigen (HBsAg), and anti-hepatitis C virus antibody (HCV)]. She then underwent renal biopsy.

Renal biopsy report revealed
- *Light microscopy*:
  - *Glomerulus*:
    - Size: Mildly enlarged
    - Cellularity: Focal mild proliferation of mesangial cells in some glomeruli.
    - Matrix: Increased (+)
    - Glomerular basement membrane (GBM): Not thick
    - Sclerosis, Crescent- 0
  - *Tubules*:
    - Epithelium: Features of protein reabsorption
    - Cast: Hyaline
  - *Interstitium*:
    - Inflammation: Focal, mild, and chronic
  - *Blood vessels*:
    - Unremarkable

- *Direct immunofluorescence (DIF)*:
  - ○ No deposition of any antibody is seen.
- *Comment*:
  - ○ Minimal change disease

She was prescribed oral prednisolone (1 mg/kg/day) and it was continued for 16 weeks. UTP came down to 4 g/day. She was then switched to oral cyclosporine 3.5 mg/kg/day with low-dose prednisolone 10 mg/day and it was continued for 1 year with stable proteinuria (UTP 4.3 g/day). After that, she discontinued treatment by herself. 4 months later, she was again put on oral cyclosporine 3.5 mg/kg/day with oral prednisolone 10 mg/day. After continuing treatment for 2 months, she developed generalized swelling with reduced urine output and was found to have renal impairment with a rise of serum creatinine up to 9 mg/dL. She received three doses of injection methylprednisolone followed by oral prednisolone 1 mg/kg/day. She undergone few sessions of hemodialysis. Renal function became normal. Renal histopathology slide was reviewed.

Review report revealed:
- *Glomerulus*:
  - ○ Mild increase of mesangial cells and matrix
  - ○ Two of these glomeruli show segmental sclerosis
  - ○ GBM: Mildly irregular thick
- *Tubules*:
  - ○ Tubular epithelium: Abundant eosinophilic granular cytoplasm
  - ○ Cast: Hyaline
- *Interstitium*:
  - ○ Focal infiltration of chronic inflammatory cells and mild fibrosis
- *Blood vessels*:
  - ○ Mildly thick-walled
- *Comment*:
  - ○ Possibility of focal segmental glomerulosclerosis (FSGS) may be considered.

Based on this report, she was started on high-dose dexamethasone 0.9 mg/kg with mycophenolate mofetil (MMF) 2 g/day. Treatment was continued for 4 months without any remission (UTP 8 g/day) and 1 month after discontinuation of treatment, her UTP rose to 12 g/day and serum creatinine started to rise. She was treated with antiproteinuric drug over the course of her illness.

We decided to go for repeat renal biopsy. Biopsy yielded 10 glomeruli, which revealed:
- *Glomeruli*: Nine shows global sclerosis and one shows segmental sclerosis. There is mild mesangial proliferation and mild thickening of GBM, but no endocapillary proliferation, necrotizing lesion or crescent.
- *Interstitium and tubules*: Interstitial fibrosis and tubular atrophy occupied 40% of cortical area. Acute tubular injury is seen. Interstitium shows mild lymphocytic infiltration.

- *Blood vessels*: Arteries and arterioles are unremarkable.
- *DIF*: 11 glomeruli with no deposits.
- *Diagnosis*: Chronic sclerosing nephropathy with interstitial fibrosis
  Serum creatinine rose to 8 mg/dL. Other biochemical markers showed features of chronic kidney disease. Patient was adequately counseled regarding the chronic and irreversible nature of the illness. She was of renal replacement therapy.

DISCUSSION

Minimal change disease (MCD) is podocytopathy more commonly seen in children. On the other hand, idiopathic FSGS is observed in persons aged 18–45 years. The age of presentation of the patient was 19 years. The initial biopsy report was in favor of MCD. In general, adult MCD is similar to steroid sensitive nephrotic syndrome in children but the response to glucocorticoid treatment is slower in adults than in children. Approximately 10–20% of adult MCD patients are steroid resistant. Our patient was steroid resistant. One caveat is that FSGS lesions may be missed and may be misdiagnosed as MCD. And up to around 80% of cases of primary FSGS are steroid resistant. In the present case, at one point calcineurin inhibitor (CNI) was added (with low-dose steroid) but proteinuria did not come down below 4 g/day. In the natural history of a chronic glomerular disease where severe loss of kidney function is accompanied by irreversible kidney injury (interstitial fibrosis and tubular atrophy), the therapeutic options cannot alter progressive nature of deterioration of renal function which happened in our case.

FREQUENTLY ASKED QUESTIONS

Q1. What was the most likely histological diagnosis in this case?

Ans. Focal segmental glomerulosclerosis was the most likely histological diagnosis, because sometimes it happens that tissue from corticomedullary junction with focal and segmental changes may be missed in the initial biopsy.

Q2. Was it a case of steroid-resistant disease?

Ans. Yes. It was most likely a case of steroid-resistant FSGS.

Q3. How to treat steroid-resistant FSGS?

Ans. Cyclosporine or tacrolimus along with low-dose glucocorticoid may be given for ≥6 months.

Q4. What is FSGS of undetermined cause (FSGS-UC)?

Ans. FSGS can occur in absence of genetic or identifiable secondary cause, in the absence of nephrotic syndrome and without diffuse foot process effacement. This entity may be called FSGS-UC.

INDEX

Page numbers followed by *f* refer to figure and *t* refer to table.

A

Abdomen, ultrasonography of 7, 128
Abdominal examination 98
Acid-fast bacillus 47
Activated partial thromboplastin time 7, 57, 62, 101, 107
Acute kidney injury 31, 70, 75, 121
 diagnosis of 32
Adenosine triphosphate 51
Adrenal gland 79
Adult minimal change disease 62
Advanced glycation end products 3
Alanine transaminase 101, 107
Aldolase 33
Alport syndrome 72-74
Amlodipine 99
Amyloidosis 40, 125
 treatment of primary 126
Anemia 56
Angiotensin-converting enzyme 14
 inhibitor 3, 60, 64, 70
Angiotensin-receptor blocker 3, 70
Ankylosing spondylitis 35
Anorexia 1
Antibody
 antineutrophil cytoplasmic 11, 13, 17, 39
 antinuclear 10, 14, 39, 62, 73, 81, 85, 91, 101, 128
 antiphospholipid 19
 donor-specific 99
 mediated rejection 19
Anticardiolipin antibodies 19
Antiglomerular basement membrane disease 17
Antihepatitis C virus 73
Anti-human
 immunodeficiency virus 39
 leukocyte antigen 20
Antithymocyte globulin 99
Antituberculosis 13

Anuria 106
Arterial blood gas analysis 35
Arteriovenous fistula 27
Atorvastatin 62
Audiological report 74
Autosomal dominant polycystic kidney disease 112
Azathioprine 112

B

Bartter syndrome 37
Biochemical parameters 122*t*
Biochemical tests 77*t*
Biopsy report 89
Bisoprolol 89, 99
Bladder 78
 CT scan of 78
 neck incision 21
 region, ultrasonography of 62, 68*f*
 ultrasonography of 57, 68, 91, 118
Bleeding time 101, 128
Blood
 biochemistry 24
 count 28*t*
 film, peripheral 78, 91
 pressure 1, 7, 22, 23*t*, 26, 56, 61, 66, 113
 sugar, random 73, 91, 101, 107
 vessel 53, 82, 86
Body mass index 27
Bone marrow examination 78
 report 40, 129
Bone tissue 129
Brain, MRI of 8, 8*f*

C

Calcineurin inhibitor 133
 post-transplant 18
Calcium acetate 89
Carbonyl iron 89
Cardiovascular risk reduction 3

Cellular rejection 97
  diagnosis of acute 104
Chemoprophylaxis 118
Chest
  CT scan of 94f
  noncontrast CT scan of 8
  X-ray 14, 62, 78
Cholecalciferol 89
Chronic kidney disease 1, 3, 18, 21, 26,
  43, 46, 75, 88, 97, 105, 112, 115, 133
Clotting time 101, 128
Cold ischemic time 26
Collagenofibrotic glomerulopathy 88,
  91
Complete blood count 2, 28, 57, 62, 68,
  73, 73t, 78, 100t, 106t, 116t, 122t, 128t
Computed tomography 35, 47
Concentric left ventricular hypertrophy
  125
Congo-red stain 40
Continuous ambulatory peritoneal
  dialysis 4, 46
  peritonitis 46
Cortical echogenicity 73
Corticomedullary differentiation 44,
  73, 129
Corticosteroids 83
Cotrimoxazole 97
COVID-19
  vaccination 88
  vaccine 92
C-reactive protein 77, 101, 117
  high-sensitivity 107
Creatine kinase 33
Cyclophosphamide 16
  intravenous 16
Cytomegalovirus 18, 26, 28, 93, 99, 101,
  112
  infection 95
  pneumonia 93
Cytoplasmic antineutrophil cytoplasmic
  antibodies 13, 57, 73, 85, 91, 101,
  128

D

Dense deposit disease 59
Diabetes mellitus 35
  post-transplant 26
Diabetic foot ulcer 2f
Diabetic nephropathy 1, 3

Diabetic proliferative retinopathy 2f
Diazepam, intramuscular 6
Dimercaptosuccinic acid 44, 111
Direct immunofluorescence 53, 58, 59t,
  64t, 69, 82, 86, 123, 125, 132
Dithiothreitol 21
Domperidone 89
Doppler imaging 101
Doppler ultrasonography 108
Down's syndrome 43
Dry cough 13

E

Echocardiography 3
Ejection fraction 7
Endocapillary proliferation 81
Epithelium 8, 86
Erythrocyte sedimentation rate 2, 7, 57,
  68, 73, 78, 91, 100, 106, 116, 122, 128
Erythropoiesis-stimulating agent 3
Erythropoietin 89
Estimated glomerular filtration rate 3,
  86, 116
Ethambutol 76

F

Famotidine 62
Febuxostat 76, 89
Femoral head, avascular necrosis of 81
Ferritin 73
Fibrin degradation product 18
Fibrosis 86
Flucloxacillin 76
Focal lymphocytic infiltration 82
Focal segmental
  deposition 53
  glomerulosclerosis 49, 50, 50f, 51, 51f,
  53, 62, 131
Foley's catheter, balloon of 79
Foley's urinary catheterization 76
Free light chain 41
Fundoscopic examination 74
Furosemide 62

G

Gastrointestinal survey 50
Gastrointestinal system 27
Gitelman syndrome 35, 36
Glasgow Coma Scale 124

Glomerular basement membrane 8, 57, 63, 69, 74, 82, 86, 123
Glomerular capillary wall, double contour of 81
Glomerular filtration rate 11
Glomerular tufts 40
Glomerulonephritis 11, 45, 93
  causes of 131
  diagnosis of 105
  infection-associated 70
  positive 13
  secondary causes of 53
Glomerulosclerosis, secondary focal segmental 44
Glomerulus 8, 40, 53, 57, 63, 81, 85, 132
Glyceryl trinitrate 22
Graft function 106t
Granular pattern 53
Granulomatous disease 15

H

Headache 38
Heart 124
  disease, ischemic 1
Hematologic dysfunction 114
Hematoxylin 15f
Hematuria 44, 97
Hemodialysis 46, 93
Hemoglobin 2, 19, 73, 78, 91, 100, 106
Hemolytic uremic syndrome 19
Henoch–Schönlein purpura nephritis 10, 66, 70
Hepatitis
  B core antigen 91
  B virus 72
  C virus 19, 28, 101
Herpesvirus 19
High power field 1, 7, 31, 38, 44, 49, 57, 62, 67, 100, 121
Hip joint
  MRI of 82
  X-ray of 82, 82f, 83f
Histopathology report 129
Human immunodeficiency virus 19
Human leukocyte antigen 99, 117
  typing 105t
Hydroureteronephrosis, bilateral 21
Hydroxyurea 130
Hypertension 26, 35, 46, 53, 93, 105
Hypocalciuria 36, 37
Hypochloremia 35

Hypokalemia 35-37
Hypokinesia 3
Hypomagnesemia 35-37

I

Idiopathic thrombocytopenic purpura 76
Imipenem 76
Immunization, expanded programme on 7, 66
Immunofluorescence 40, 50
Immunoglobulin
  A 10, 59, 123
    vasculitis 67
  G 59, 60, 86, 93, 99, 123
  M 28, 50, 53, 59, 99, 123
    nephropathy 53, 54
Infarcts, acute 8
Inflammation 58, 86
  chronic, mild 8
  mild and chronic 64
Inflammatory cells, chronic 58
Influenza 72
  A 19
Intact parathyroid hormone 73, 77, 91, 107
Intensive care unit 33, 43
Interstitial fibrosis 82
Interstitium 8, 40, 53, 58, 64, 82, 86, 132

J

Joints, pain in multiple 6
Jugular venous pressure 27, 56, 61, 66, 124

K

Kayser–Fleischer ring 50
Kidney 62, 124, 129
  biopsy 40
    report, transplanted 103
  computed tomography of 78
  CT scan of 78
  disease, end-stage 3
  left 79
  right 78
  transplant 29, 93
  ultrasonography of 57, 62, 68, 68f, 91, 118

L

Laboratory investigations 90*t*
Laboratory parameters 100*t*, 107*t*, 116*t*
Lactate dehydrogenase 31, 107
Leg swelling
  bilateral 13
  redness, and blackish area on 113*f*
Leukocytoclastic vasculitis 70
Leukonychia 56
Levothyroxine sodium 89
Light microscopic examination 57, 63
Lipomyelomeningocele 75, 79
Lipoprotein
  high-density 2, 28, 57, 91
  low-density 2, 28, 57, 91, 101
Liver 27
Lobar collapse 15*f*
Lobular accentuation 81
Lower limb 67*f*
Lower urinary tract abnormality 21
Lupus nephritis 6, 62, 70, 81, 120
  class 10*f*
Lymphocytic infiltration, mild 132

M

Malignancy 19
Masson's trichrome 40
Mean corpuscular hemoglobin 57, 116
Mechanical ventilation 114
Membranoproliferative
  glomerulonephritis 56
  periodic acid-Schiff 58*f*
Membranous nephropathy 61, 62, 63*f*,
  64, 85, 86, 91
Mesangial proliferative
  glomerulonephritis 53, 62
Methylprednisolone, intravenous 18
Microscopic appearance 103
Microscopic description 40
Microscopy
  electron 89
  light 69*t*, 125
Microvascular thrombi 19
Micturating cystourethrogram 44
Miliary lung lesion 78*f*
Minimal change disease 91, 131, 133
Mitral regurgitation, mild 125
Mycobacterium tuberculosis 47

Mycophenolate mofetil 97, 121
Mycophenolic acid 93
Myelodysplastic syndrome 127
Myoglobinuria 32

N

Nausea 1
Necrotizing sarcoid granuloma 16
Nephritic urinary sediment 16
Nephropathy 50
  treatment of 129
Nephrotic syndrome 51, 70, 85, 127, 128
Nephrotoxic medications 127
Neurogenic bladder 75
Neutrophils 46
Nifedipine 89
Nocturnal dyspnea 124
Noncytotoxic agents 130
Nonsteroidal anti-inflammatory drugs
  31, 85
Nucleic acid test 95

O

Obstructive uropathy-neurogenic
  bladder 118
Oral mycophenolate mofetil 49

P

Parathyroid hormone 116
Parenchyma 118
Parvovirus B$_{19}$ 19
Perinuclear antineutrophil cytoplasmic
  antibody 62, 68, 73, 85, 101, 128
Periodic acid-Schiff 40, 63*f*
Periodic Schiff-methenamine 40
Peritoneal dialysis 4
  catheter 47
Peritonitis 47
Phenytoin, intravenous 6
Plasma cells 40
Pleural effusion, bilateral 124
Pneumococcus 72
Polyangiitis, granulomatosis with 15
Polymerase chain reaction 101
Ponticelli regimen, modified 62
Positive perinuclear antineutrophil
  cytoplasmic antibody 81
Positron emission tomography 13

Potassium supplementation 37
Prazosin 89, 99
Prednisolone 89, 99, 132
Proliferative diabetic retinopathy 1
Proliferative lupus nephritis, diffuse 82
Prostate 79
Protein
    kinase C, activation of 3
    reabsorption 8
Proteinuria 44, 51, 97
Prothrombin time 68, 101, 107, 128
Puffy face 56
Pulmonary tuberculosis 27
Pus cell 67
Pyelonephritis, chronic 118, 115
Pyrazinamide 76

R

Rabeprazole 89
Ramipril 62
Randomized controlled trial 86
Rash 66
Recipient and donor workup 99t
Red blood cell 7, 14, 44, 46, 57, 67, 69,
    83, 100, 116, 121, 123, 127
Red cell
    cast 81
    concentrates 106
Reflux nephropathy 118
Refractory lupus nephritis 120
Renal abscess 115
Renal allograft recipient 97, 112
Renal amyloidosis 38
Renal angiogram, computed
    tomography 109
Renal biopsy 8, 18, 40, 120
    report 57, 63, 69, 122t, 131
Renal disease
    end-stage 44, 74, 93
    modification of 35
Renal dysplasia 118
Renal failure, acute 31
Renal function test 73, 73t, 100t, 116t,
    122t
Renal impairment 46
Renal injury 51
Renal parenchymal disease, bilateral 73
Renal replacement therapy 26, 44, 46

Renal transplant 75, 114
Renal transplantation
    pre-emptive 26
    vascular complication after 105
Renin-angiotensin-aldosterone system 3
Respiratory rate 56
Respiratory system 98
    examination of 27
Respiratory tract 16
Rhabdomyolysis 32
Rimactazid 76
Rituximab 16, 130

S

Sclerosis 63
Sepsis 112
Serological tests 117t
Serum 100
    albumin 57, 73
    calcium 73
    creatinine 68, 77
    electrolytes 68, 77
    free light chains 39t
    glutamic pyruvic transaminase 28,
        57, 91, 107
    phosphate 73
    urea 68
    uric acid 73
Skin biopsy report 69
Slit-lamp examination 74
Sodium bicarbonate 99
Spleen 27
Stable angina, chronic 46
Stable proteinuria 132
Subendothelial widening, severe 19
Sugar 47
Swelling 1
    generalized 61
Systemic amyloidosis 124
Systemic lupus erythematosus 10, 81,
    83, 120

T

Tacrolimus 29, 99
Telmisartan 89
Tethered cord syndrome 75
Thrombotic microangiopathy 19
    post-transplant 18, 19

Thrombotic thrombocytopenic purpura 19
Thyroid-stimulating hormone 73
Toes, clawing of 77*f*
Total cholesterol 57
Total iron binding capacity 2, 29, 77, 91, 107
Transferrin saturation 7, 29, 73, 107
Transplant kidney
  color Doppler of 102
  CT renal angiogram of 110*f*
  Doppler ultrasonography of 101
  ultrasonography of 102*f*
Trephine biopsy 129
Tricuspid regurgitation 125
Tuberculosis 7, 75
  disseminated 75
Tuberculous meningitis 58, 103
Tubular atrophy 8, 58, 81, 133
Tubular basement membrane 8, 86
Tubular injury, acute 81
Tubule 40, 53, 58, 64, 81, 132
  distal convoluted 36
Tubulointerstitial nephritis 92, 129

U

Ulcer, nonhealing 1
Ultrasonography 29
Upper gastrointestinal endoscopy 50
Ureter 78, 118
  CT scan of 78
  ultrasonography of 57, 62, 68, 68*t*, 91, 118
Urinalysis 27*t*, 121*t*, 127*t*

Urinary bladder 79
Urinary total
  protein 13, 49, 53, 57, 62, 67, 73, 77, 82, 85, 100, 121, 131
  volume 67, 100, 121, 125
Urinary tract infection 21, 38, 75, 115
Urine 27, 49
  albumin to creatinine ratio 2
  dark red color 67*f*
  output 23*t*
  protein 81
  test 100*t*
  volume 85
Uroflowmetry 117*f*

V

Valganciclovir 97
Vasculitis 17
  necrotizing 16
Vesicoureteric reflux 115, 118
Vessels 40
Viral infections 19
Viral markers 28*t*
Visual acuity 72

W

Warm ischemic time 26
Wegener's granulomatosis 15
White blood cell 1, 7, 31, 46, 73, 100, 122, 128
  total count 78
Wilson's disease 49, 50, 52
Wire loop lesion 81

EU GSPR Authorised Reprsentative
Logos Europe, 9 rue Nicolas Poussin
1700, La Rochelle, France
Phone: +33 (0) 6 67 93 73 78
E-mail: contact@logoseurope.eu

www.ingramcontent.com/pod-product-compliance
Ingram Content Group UK Ltd.
Pitfield, Milton Keynes, MK11 3LW, UK
UKHW051420270526
12721UKWH00014B/1131